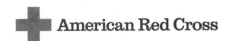

American Red Cross

# CPR FOR THE PROFESSIONAL RESCUER

## Important certification information

American Red Cross certificates may be issued upon successful completion of a training program that uses this textbook as an integral part of the course. By itself, the text material does not constitute comprehensive Red Cross training. In order to issue ARC certificates, your instructor must be authorized by the American Red Cross and must follow prescribed policies and procedures. Make certain that you have attended a course authorized by the Red Cross. Ask your instructor about receiving American Red Cross certification, or contact your local chapter for more information.

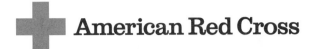

# American Red Cross

# CPR FOR THE
# PROFESSIONAL RESCUER

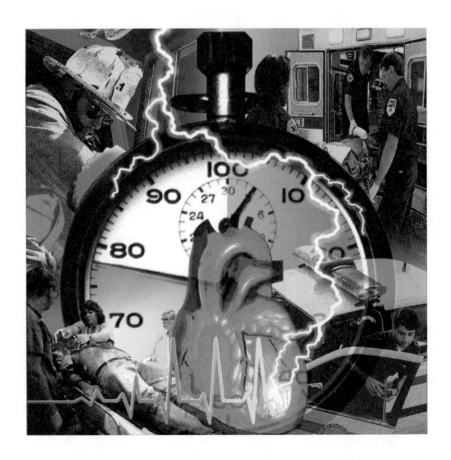

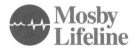

Mosby
Lifeline

St. Louis  Baltimore  Boston  Chicago  London  Philadelphia  Sydney  Toronto

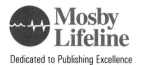

Mosby
Lifeline
Dedicated to Publishing Excellence

Printed in the United States of America

Mosby Lifeline
Mosby—Year Book, Inc.
11830 Westline Industrial Drive
St. Louis, MO 63146

**Library of Congress Cataloging in Publication Data**
CPR for the professional rescuer / American Red Cross.
     p.  cm.
    Includes index.
    ISBN (invalid) 0-8016-7067-5
    1. CPR (First aid)   I. American Red Cross.
RC87.9.C75   1993                                92-41664
616.1'025—dc20                              CIP

97  98  99  00  CL/CD/BA  9  8

# Acknowledgements

This course and participant's manual were developed and produced through a joint effort of the American Red Cross and the Mosby–Year Book Publishing Company. Many individuals shared in the overall process in many supportive, technical, and creative ways. This book could not have been developed without the dedication of both paid and volunteer staff. Their commitment to excellence made this book possible.

The Health and Safety Program Development Team at American Red Cross national headquarters responsible for the developing, designing, and writing of this course and textbook included: Lawrence D. Newell, Ed.D., NREMT-P, project manager, writer, instructional designer; S. Elizabeth White, M.A.Ed., ATC, writer, instructional designer, art and design director; Martha F. Beshers; Thomas J.S. Edwards, Ph.D.; M. Elizabeth Buoy-Morrissey, M.P.H.; Robert T. Ogle, associates; Sandra D. Buesking, Lori M. Compton, Marian F.H. Kirk, and O. Paul Stearns, analysts. Administrative support was provided by Denise Beale and Ella Holloway.

The following American Red Cross national headquarters Health and Safety volunteer and paid staff provided guidance and review: Robert F. Burnside, director; Frank Carroll, deputy regional executive officer, Mid-Atlantic Regional Office; Susan J. White, marketing specialist; Kathleen Cole Oberlin, senior associate, Operations; Stephen Silverman, Ed.D., national volunteer consultant, Health and Safety.

The Mosby Lifeline Production team based in Hanover, Maryland included: David Culverwell, vice president and publisher; Richard Weimer, executive editor; Claire Merrick, senior editor; and Dana Battaglia, assistant editor. The Mosby–Year Book editorial and production team included: Virgil Mette, executive vice president; Kay Kramer, director of art and design; Jerry A. Wood, director of manufacturing; Patricia Stinecipher, special product manager; Kathy Grone, manufacturing supervisor; Karen Edwards, project manager; Cindy Miller, senior production editor; and John Rokusek, designer.

Special thanks go to Rick Brady, photographer.

Guidance and review were also provided by the members of the
American Red Cross CPR/First Aid Advisory Group:

**Ray Cranston,**
Chairperson,
Commanding Officer, Traffic
 Safety Unit,
Farmington Hills Police
 Department,
Farmington Hills, Michigan

**Larry Bair,**
Director, Health and Safety and
 Tissue Services,
Central Iowa Chapter,
Des Moines, Iowa

**John E. Hendrickson,**
Director, Safety and Health,
Mid-America Chapter,
Chicago, Illinois

**Andra Jones,**
Director, Health and Safety,
Central Mississippi Chapter,
Jackson, Mississippi

**Sherri Olson-Roberts,**
Director, Health and Safety,
Washtenaw County Chapter,
Ann Arbor, Michigan

**James A. Otte,**
Chairman, Health and Safety
 Committee,
Glynn County Chapter,
Brunswick, Georgia

**Teresita B. Ramirez,**
Centrex County Chapter,
Lecturer, Department of
 Curriculum and Instruction,
The University of Texas at
 Austin,
Austin, Texas

**W. Douglas Round,**
Captain, Greeley Fire
 Department,
Colorado Territory,
Greeley, Colorado

**Natalie Lynne Smith, MS,**
Greater Hartford Chapter,
Farmington, Connecticut

**Linda S. Wenger,**
Director, Health and Safety,
Lancaster County Chapter,
Lancaster, Pennsylvania

**David J. Wurzer, PhD,**
Greater Long Beach Chapter,
Long Beach, California

**Frank P. Cooley, EMT-P,**
Subcommittee Chairperson,
Coordinator—EMS,
City of Des Moines Fire
 Department,
Des Moines, Iowa

**Pamela D. Alesky, R-EMT,**
Health Services Director,
Greater Erie County Chapter,
American Red Cross,
Erie, Pennsylvania

**Carol L. Belmont, RN, BES,**
Consultant,
Organization Dynamics, Inc.,
Burlington, Massachusetts

**Ricky Davidson, EMT-P,**
Chief of EMS,
Shreveport Fire Department,
Shreveport, Louisiana

**Rodney L. Dennison, EMT-P,**
EMS Program Manager,
Texas Department of Health,
Region I,
Temple, Texas

**Lance J. Kohn, Sr., EMT-P,**
Coordinator/Senior Instructor,
Town of Tonawanda Police
 Department,
Tonawanda, New York

**David W. Lewis,**
Safety Services Director,
Dallas Area Chapter,
American Red Cross,
Dallas, Texas

**Rafael A. Ortiz, EMT-P,**
Fire Fighter,
Los Angeles County Fire
 Department,
Long Beach, California

External review was provided by the following organizations:

American College of Emergency Physicians—Dallas, Texas
International Association of Fire Fighters—Washington, D.C.
National Association of EMS Physicians—Pittsburgh, Pennsylvania
National Association of Emergency Medical Technicians—
     Kansas City, Missouri
National Athletic Trainers Association—Dallas, Texas
National Council of State EMS Training Coordinators—
     Lexington, Kentucky
United States Air Force Pararescue Association—
     Albuquerque, New Mexico

External review was provided by the following individuals:

**Robert S. Behnke, HSD,**
Professor of Physical Education,
Indiana State University,
Terre Haute, Indiana

**John L. Beckman, EMT-P,**
Fire Fighter,
Lincolnwood Fire Department,
Lincolnwood, Illinois

**Clinton L. Buchanan,**
Chief, EMS Bureau,
Memphis Fire Department,
Memphis, Tennessee

**John J. Clair,**
National Ski Patrol System Inc.,
Albany, New York

**Rod Compton, MEd, ATC,**
Sports Medicine Director,
Assistant Professor,
Sports Medicine Division,
East Carolina University,
Greenville, North Carolina

**John Doyle, RN,**
EMS Coordinator,
Victor Valley Community
     College,
Victorville, California

**Richard M. Duffy,**
Director, Occupational Health
     and Safety,
International Association of Fire
     Fighters, AFL-CIO, CLC,
Washington, D.C.

**Robert Elling, NREMT-P,**
Associate Director,
New York State EMS Program,
Albany, New York

**Technical Sergeant Mark D.
     Fowler,**
Pararescue Medical Instructor,
USAF Pararescue School,
Kirtland AFB, New Mexico

**Joseph J. Godek, MS, ATC,**
West Chester University,
West Chester, Pennsylvania

**Paul Grace,**
Coordinator, Sports Medicine,
Massachusetts Institute of
     Technology,
Cambridge, Massachusetts

**Daniel F. Harshbarger, PA,**
Baltimore Gas & Electric
     Company,
Baltimore, Maryland

**Karla Holmes,**
National Council of State EMS
     Training Coordinators,
Lexington, Kentucky

**Steven A. Meador, MD,**
Assistant Professor of Medicine,
Pennsylvania State University,
The Milton S. Hershey Medical
     Center,
Hershey, Pennsylvania

**Ray Mitchell,**
EMS Director,
Trenholm State Technical
     College,
Montgomery, Alabama

**Major James K. Nickerson,**
Medical Training Advisor,
USAF Pararescue School,
Kirtland AFB, New Mexico

**Art T. Otto, NREMT-P,**
Operations Manager,
Murphy Ambulance Service Inc.,
St. Cloud, Minnesota

**James O. Page, JD,**
Publisher,
Jems Communication Inc.,
Carlsbad, California

**S. Scott Polsky, MD, FACEP,**
Member, ACEP EMS Committee,
EMS Director,
Akron City Hospital,
Akron, Ohio

**David C. Pryor, MSM, EMT-P,**
EMS Department Chairperson,
Associate Professor—Senior,
Miami Dade Community
     College,
Miami, Florida

**Barbara Reisbach,**
Coordinator, Public Safety
     Service,
EHOVE Career Center,
Vanguard—Sentinel JVS,
Fremont, Ohio

**Matthew M. Rice, MD, JD,**
Chairman and Program Director,
Department of Emergency
  Medicine,
Madigan Army Medical Center,
Fort Lewis, Washington

**Paul D. Roman, REMT,**
Chairman, ASTM F30.02.03 Task
  Group on First Responders,
Executive Director,
New Jersey EMT Registry,
Shrewsbury, New Jersey

**Sergeant James Shelly, RN,**
First Responder Instructor,
Baltimore Police Department,
Children's Hospital of Baltimore,
Baltimore, Maryland

**James P. Shinners,**
Director, Health Service,
American Red Cross,
St. Paul Area Chapter,
St. Paul, Minnesota

**Sherman K. Sowby, PhD,
  CHES,**
Professor of Health Science,
California State University at
  Fresno,
Fresno, California

**Mary Ann Talley,**
Program Director,
EMS Education,
University of South Alabama,
Mobile, Alabama

**Bill Vargas,**
President,
USAF Pararescue Association,
Albuquerque, New Mexico

**Gary W. Waites, EMT-P, EMSC,**
EMS Course Coordinator,
College of the Mainland,
Emergency Response
  Coordinator,
Amoco Corporation,
Alvin, Texas

**Master Sergeant Edward C.
  Washburn,**
USAF EMT Program Manager,
3790th Medical Service Training
  Wing,
Sheppard AFB, Texas

**Gene Weatherall,**
Chief,
Bureau of Emergency
  Management,
Texas Department of Health,
Austin, Texas

**Katherine H. West, BSN,
  MSEd, CIC,**
Consultant,
Infection Control/Emerging
  Concepts Inc.,
Springfield, Virginia

**Michael D. Zemany, AEMT/3,**
Deputy Director,
North County Community
  College,
Mt. Lakes Regional EMS
  Programs,
Saranac Lake, New York

# Contents

# Detailed Table of Contents

# About This Course

## ◆ WHY YOU SHOULD TAKE THIS COURSE

It would be ideal if everyone knew what to do when suddenly confronted with an emergency. But that is not reality. Instead, people tend to look to others who are more knowledgeable about what care to provide to an injured or ill person. You, the professional rescuer, are often the first trained person to arrive at the emergency scene. You will be expected to take appropriate action to provide care for injuries or sudden illnesses until more advanced medical personnel arrive. This course prepares you to fulfill this role as a professional rescuer.

## ◆ HOW YOU WILL LEARN

Course content is presented in various ways. Video segments present information and skills that are then discussed in class. Course participants practice these skills. These video segments emphasize the key points you need to remember when making decisions in emergencies and help you provide the proper care. This participant's manual contains the information and skills provided in the video segments.

The course design allows you to frequently evaluate your progress in terms of skills com-

petency, knowledge, and decision-making. Your ability to correctly perform specific skills shown in the video and described in the participant's manual will be checked by your instructor during practice sessions. Your ability to make appropriate decisions when faced with an emergency will be enhanced as you participate in various class activities.

Periodically, you will be given situations in the form of scenarios that provide you the opportunity to apply the knowledge and skills you have learned. These scenarios also provide an opportunity to discuss with your instructor and classmates the many different situations that you may encounter in any emergency.

## ◆ REQUIREMENTS FOR COURSE COMPLETION CERTIFICATE

When this course is taught by a currently authorized American Red Cross instructor, you will be eligible for an American Red Cross course completion certificate. In order for you to receive an American Red Cross course completion certificate, you must—

- ◆ Perform specific skills competently and demonstrate the ability to make appropriate decisions for care.

- Pass a final written examination with a score of 80% or higher.

The final written examination is designed to test your retention and understanding of the course material. You will take this examination at the end of the course. If you do not pass this examination the first time, you may take a second examination.

## ◆ PARTICIPANT'S MANUAL

This participant's manual has been designed to facilitate your learning and understanding of the material it presents. It includes the following features:

## Objectives

At the beginning of each chapter is a list of objectives. Read these objectives carefully and refer back to them from time to time as you read the chapter. The objectives describe what you should be able to do after reading the chapter and participating in class activities.

## Key Terms

After the objectives is a list of defined key terms you need to know to understand chapter content. The pronunciation of certain medical and anatomical terms is provided, and a pronunciation guide is included in the glossary. In the chapter, key terms are printed in bold type the first time they are defined or explained.

## Main Ideas

A section called "Main Ideas" follows the key terms. These are the major concepts in the chapter and each is expressed in one or two sentences.

## Sidebars

Feature articles called sidebars appear in certain chapters and enhance the content of the main body of the text. They present a variety of material ranging from historical information and accounts of actual events to everyday application of the information presented in the main body of the text. You will not be tested on any information presented in these sidebars as part of the American Red Cross course completion requirements.

## Tables

Tables are included in many chapters. They concisely summarize important concepts and information and may aid in studying.

## Review Questions

At the end of each chapter are a series of multiple-choice questions designed to test your retention and understanding of the material in the chapter. Answers to the questions are in small print at the bottom of the page.

## Skill Sheets

Skill sheets at the end of certain chapters provide you with step-by-step, illustrated directions for performing certain skills described in the chapter and shown on the video.

## Appendix

One appendix at the end of this textbook provides additional information on a topic professional rescuers will find useful. The subject is automated external defibrillation.

## Glossary

The glossary includes definitions of all the key terms and of other words in the text that may be unfamiliar. A pronunciation guide is included in the glossary. All glossary terms appear in the textbook in bold type.

# Health Precautions and Guidelines for the Professional Rescuer

The American Red Cross has trained millions of people in first aid and CPR (cardiopulmonary resuscitation) using manikins as training aids. According to the Centers for Disease Control (CDC), there has never been a documented case of any disease caused by bacteria, a fungus, or a virus transmitted through the use of training aids such as manikins used for CPR.

The Red Cross follows widely accepted guidelines for cleaning and decontaminating training manikins. **If these guidelines are adhered to, the risk of any kind of disease transmission during training is extremely low.**

To help minimize the risk of disease transmission, you should follow some basic health precautions and guidelines while participating in training. You should take precautions if you have a condition that would increase your risk or other participants' risk of exposure to infections. Request a separate training manikin if you—

+ Have an acute condition, such as a cold, a sore throat, or cuts or sores on your hands or around your mouth.

+ Know you are seropositive (have had a positive blood test) for hepatitis B surface antigen (HBsAg), indicating that you are currently infected with the hepatitis B virus.*
+ Know you have a chronic infection indicated by long-term seropositivity (long-term positive blood tests) for the hepatitis B surface antigen (HBsAg)* or a positive blood test for anti-HIV (that is, a positive test for antibodies to HIV, the virus that causes many severe infections including AIDS).

*A person with hepatitis B infection will test positive for the hepatitis B surface antigen (HBsAg). Most persons infected with hepatitis B will get better within a period of time. However, some hepatitis B infections will become chronic and will linger for much longer. These persons will continue to test positive for HBsAg. Their decision to participate in CPR training should be guided by their physician.*

*After a person has had an acute hepatitis B infection, he or she will no longer test positive for the surface antigen but will test positive for the hepatitis B antibody (anti-HBs). Persons who have been vaccinated for hepatitis B will also test positive for the hepatitis antibody. A positive test for the hepatitis B antibody (anti-HBs) should not be confused with a positive test for the hepatitis B surface antigen (HBsAg).*

◆ Have a type of condition that makes you unusually likely to get an infection.

**If you decide you should have your own manikin, ask your instructor if he or she can provide one for you to use.** You will not be asked to explain why in your request. The manikin will not be used by anyone else until it has been cleaned according to the recommended end-of-class decontamination procedures. Because the number of manikins available for class use is limited, the more advance notice you give, the more likely it is that you can be provided a separate manikin.

In addition to taking the precautions regarding manikins, you can further protect yourself and other participants from infection by following these guidelines:

◆ Wash your hands thoroughly before participating in class activities.
◆ Do not eat, drink, use tobacco products, or chew gum during classes when manikins are used.

◆ Clean the manikin properly before use. For some manikins, this means vigorously wiping the manikin's face and the inside of its mouth with a clean gauze pad soaked with either a solution of liquid chlorine bleach and water (sodium hypochlorite and water) or rubbing alcohol. For other manikins, it means changing the rubber face. Your instructor will provide you with instructions for cleaning the type of manikin used in your class.
◆ Follow the guidelines provided by your instructor when practicing skills such as clearing a blocked airway with your finger.

## ◆ PHYSICAL STRESS AND INJURY

Training in first aid and CPR requires physical activity. If you have a medical condition or disability that will prevent you from taking part in the practice sessions, please let your instructor know.

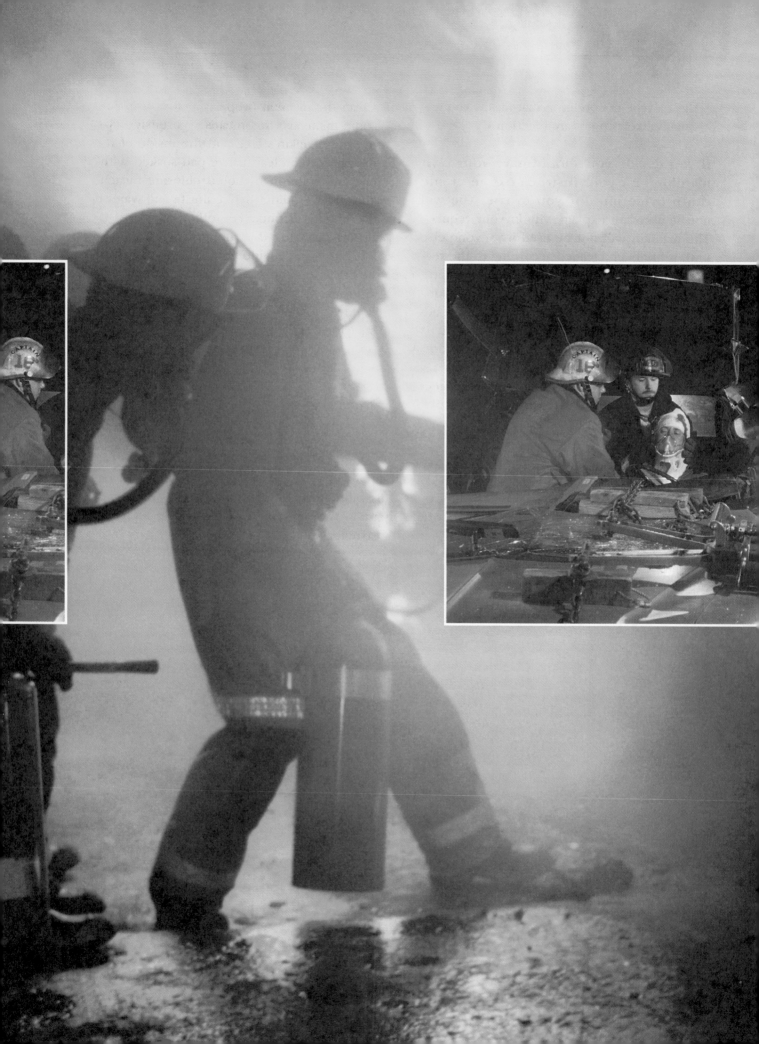

# Part One

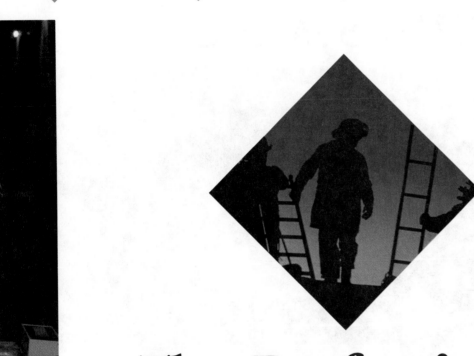

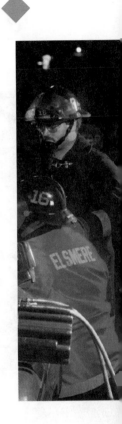

# The Professional Rescuer

1

The Professional Rescuer and the EMS System

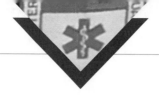

# The Professional Rescuer and the EMS System

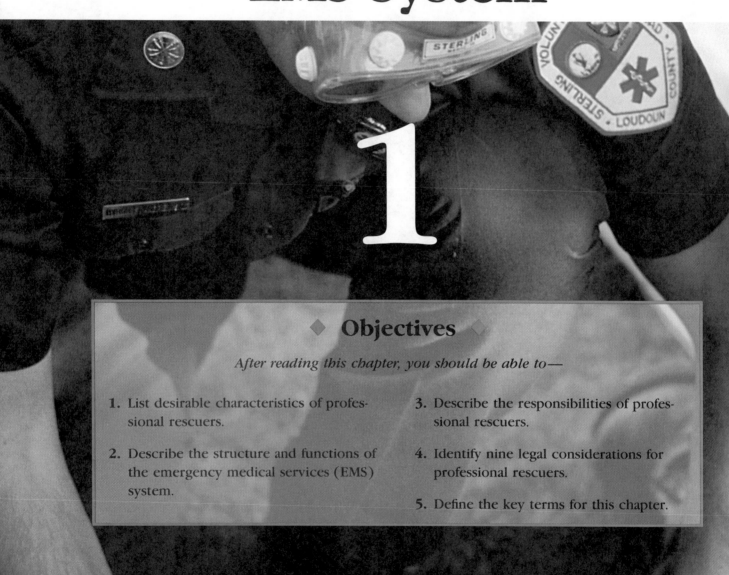

## ◆ Objectives ◆

*After reading this chapter, you should be able to—*

1. List desirable characteristics of professional rescuers.

2. Describe the structure and functions of the emergency medical services (EMS) system.

3. Describe the responsibilities of professional rescuers.

4. Identify nine legal considerations for professional rescuers.

5. Define the key terms for this chapter.

## ◆ Key Terms ◆

**Abandonment:** Ending care of an ill or injured person without that person's consent or without ensuring that someone with equal or greater training will continue care.

**Confidentiality:** Protecting a victim's privacy by not revealing any personal information you learn about the victim except to law enforcement personnel or EMS personnel caring for the victim.

**Consent:** Permission to provide care, given by an ill or injured person to a rescuer.

**Duty to act:** A legal responsibility of certain people to provide a reasonable standard of emergency care; may be required by case law, statute, or job description.

**Emergency medical services (EMS) system:** A network of community resources and personnel that provides emergency care to victims of injury or sudden illness.

**Emergency medical technician (EMT):** Someone who has successfully completed a state-approved Emergency Medical Technical training program. Different levels of EMTs exist: paramedics, for example, are at the highest level.

**Good Samaritan laws:** Laws that protect people who willingly give emergency care without accepting anything in return.

**Negligence:** The failure to provide the level of care a person of similar training would provide, thereby causing injury or damage to another.

**Refusal of care:** The declining of care by a victim; a victim bears the right to refuse the care of anyone who responds to an emergency scene.

**Standard of care:** The minimal standard and quality of care expected of an emergency care provider.

## ◆ Main Ideas ◆

1. Professional rescuers serve their communities in many ways, but they share specific characteristics and responsibilities.
2. The professional rescuer is a critical link in the emergency medical services (EMS) system—a link in the chain of survival.
3. The professional rescuer should be aware of certain legal considerations governing care.

## ◆ THE PROFESSIONAL RESCUER

As a professional rescuer, you are a key part of the emergency medical services (EMS) system. Whether paid or volunteer, you are summoned to provide care in an emergency. Unlike a layperson, you have a professional duty to act in an emergency and give care. Your actions are often critical. They may determine whether a seriously ill or injured person survives. To provide appropriate emergency care, you must gain adequate knowledge, skills, and confidence.

This course is designed for those people who have been or who are being trained to assume responsibilities for delivering health care and/or ensuring public safety. The roles of people who work as professional rescuers are varied and include the following:

- Allied health professionals (for example, medical assistants, physical therapists, respiratory therapists, and X-ray technicians)
- Athletic trainers

- Business and industry personnel
- Emergency medical technicians (EMTs)
- Fire fighters
- Flight attendants
- Law enforcement personnel
- Lifeguards
- Members of search and rescue teams
- Nurses
- Paramedics
- Park rangers
- Physicians
- Public safety personnel
- Security personnel
- Ski patrollers

## Responsibilities

Although professional rescuers have many different occupations, you share important responsibilities that include—

- A duty, when on the job, to respond to an emergency.
- Using certain techniques that require professional training and are not generally taught to the lay public.
- Ensuring personal safety and bystander safety.
- Gaining access to the victim.
- Determining any threats to the victim's life.
- Providing needed care for the victim.
- Summoning more appropriate personnel when necessary.

## Personal Characteristics

As someone who deals with the public, you must be willing to take on responsibilities beyond giving care. These responsibilities require you to demonstrate certain characteristics that include—

- *Maintaining a caring and professional attitude.* Ill or injured people are sometimes difficult to work with. Be compassionate; try to understand their concerns and fears. Realize that any anger they may show is often the result of fear. Lay people who help during the emergency may also be afraid.

Try to be reassuring. Even though they may not have done everything perfectly, be sure to thank them for taking action. Recognition and praise affirm their willingness to act.

- *Controlling your own fears.* Try not to reveal your anxieties to the victim or bystanders. The presence of blood, vomit, or unpleasant odors is disturbing to most people. You may need to compose yourself before acting. If you must, turn away for a moment and take a few deep breaths before providing care.
- *Presenting a professional appearance.* This helps ease a victim's fears and inspires confidence.
- *Keeping your skills and knowledge up to date.* Involve yourself in continuing education, professional reading, and refresher training.
- *Staying fit with daily exercise and a healthy diet.* Job stresses can adversely affect your health. Exercise and diet help manage physical, mental, and emotional stress.
- *Maintaining a safe and healthy lifestyle.* Maintaining a safe and healthy lifestyle is important both on and off the job. Completing the Healthy Heart IQ in Chapter 7 will help you identify some potential risks in your own life so that you can take steps to reduce them.

## ◆ THE EMERGENCY MEDICAL SERVICES (EMS) SYSTEM

The emergency medical services (EMS) system is a network of community resources and medical personnel that provides emergency care to victims of injury or sudden illness. When bystanders at an emergency scene recognize an emergency and take action, they activate this system. The care provided by more highly trained professionals continues until an ill or injured person receives the level of care that he or she needs.

The development of this organized EMS network over the years has led to a higher quality of medical care in our society. Thirty years ago the quality of emergency care outside the hospital was poor. Ambulance attendants only transported ill or injured people to the hospital for emergency care. Since these attendants had minimal training, ambulances were little more than fast transportation.

In 1966, the National Academy of Sciences, in a landmark paper entitled "Accidental Death and Disability: The Neglected Disease of Modern Society," brought to light the dismal quality of emergency care. The paper criticized both ambulance services and hospital emergency departments. As a result, in 1973, the United States Congress enacted the Emergency Medical Services Act. This act created a multitiered, nationwide system of emergency health care. From that start the EMS system, as we know it today, evolved. The National Highway Traffic Safety Administration (NHTSA), a division of the U.S. Department of Transportation, has supported the development of training programs for the various levels of prehospital care personnel.

## ◆ THE EMERGENCY RESPONSE—A CHAIN OF SURVIVAL

The EMS system functions as a series of events linked in a chain, a chain of survival (Fig. 1-1). The basic principle is to bring rapid medical care to the victim rather than the victim to

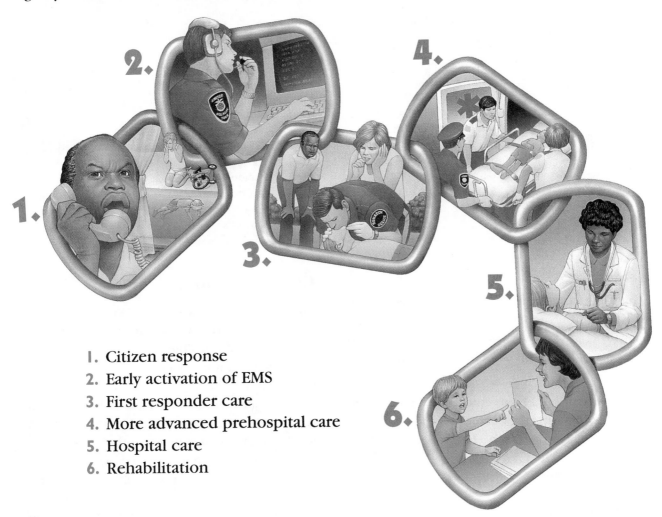

1. Citizen response
2. Early activation of EMS
3. First responder care
4. More advanced prehospital care
5. Hospital care
6. Rehabilitation

**Figure 1-1**  The Chain of Survival

# From Horses to Helicopters: A History of Emergency Care

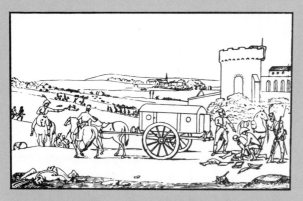

Yesterday's "Flying Ambulance" (Cabanes, Chirurgiens et Blesses a travers I' Histoire, Paris, 1918.)

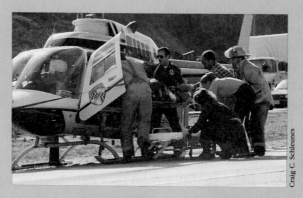

Today's "Flying Ambulance"

Emergency care originated during the French emperor Napoleon's campaigns in the late 1700s. The surgeon-in-chief for the Grand Army, Dominique Jean Larrey, became the first doctor to try to save the wounded during battles instead of waiting until the fighting was over.[1] Using horse-drawn litters, Larrey and his men dashed onto the battlefield in what became known as "flying ambulances."

By the 1860s, the wartime principles of emergency care were applied to everyday emergencies in some American cities. In 1878, a writer for *Harper's New Monthly Magazine* explained how accidents were reported to the police, who notified the nearest hospitals by a telegraph signal. He described an early hospital ambulance ride in New York City.[2]

"A well-kept horse was quickly harnessed to the ambulance; and as the surgeon took his seat behind, having first put on a jaunty uniform cap with gold lettering, the driver sprang to the box . . . and with a sharp crack of the whip we

medical care. From the onset of illness or injury until the victim receives hospital care, the survival and recovery of critically ill or injured people depends on this chain of events.

These events include—
1. Recognition of an emergency and initial care by citizen responders.
2. Early activation of the EMS system.
3. First responder care.
4. More advanced prehospital care.
5. Hospital care.
6. Rehabilitation.

## Citizen Response

The first crucial link in the EMS system is the action of the **citizen responder.** This link depends on a responsible citizen who takes action when an injury or illness occurs. This person must first recognize that what has happened is an emergency. He or she must then activate the EMS system by dialing 9-1-1 or a local 7-digit number or by notifying a nearby first responder such as a police officer.

While waiting for more highly trained personnel, the citizen responder can provide basic care to the ill or injured person. Often the

rolled off the smooth asphalt of the courtyard and into the street. . . . As we swept around corners and dashed over crossings, both doctor and driver kept up a sharp cry of warning to pedestrians."[2]

While booming industrial cities developed emergency transport systems, rural populations had only rudimentary services. In most small towns, the mortician had the only vehicle large enough to handle the litters, so emergency victims were just as likely to ride in a hearse to the hospital as in an ambulance.[3]

Cars gave Americans a faster system of transport, but over the next 50 years, car collisions also created the need for more emergency vehicles. In 1966, a major report questioned the quality of emergency services. Dismayed at the rising death toll on the nation's highways, Congress passed laws in 1966 and 1973 ordering the improved training of ambulance workers and emergency department staffs, an improved communications network, and the development of regional units with specialized care.

Today, the telegraph signal has been replaced by the 9-1-1 telephone code, which immediately connects a caller to a dispatcher who can send help. In some areas a computer connected to the enhanced 9-1-1 system displays the caller's name, address, and phone number, even if the caller cannot speak. Ambulance workers have changed from coachmen to trained medical professionals who can provide lifesaving care at the scene. Horses have been replaced by ambulances and helicopters equipped to provide the most advanced prehospital care available.

The EMS system has expanded in sheer numbers and in services. Today, New York City has 15 times as many hospitals as in the 1870s. Hospitals have also vastly improved their emergency care capabilities. If patients suffer from critical injuries, such as burns, spinal cord injuries, or other traumatic injuries, the EMS system now has developed regional trauma and burn centers where specialists are always available.

In two centuries, the EMS system has gone from horses to helicopters. As technology continues to advance, it is difficult to imagine what changes the next century will bring.

**REFERENCES**

1. Major R, M.D.: *A history of medicine,* Springfield, Ill, 1954, Charles C Thomas.
2. Rideing WH: Hospital life in New York, *Harper's New Monthly Magazine* 57:171, 1878.
3. Division of Medical Sciences, National Academy of Sciences—National Research Council: *Accidental death and disability: the neglected disease of modern society,* Washington, DC, September 1966.

care provided by citizen responders in these first few minutes is critical. However, their efforts may be futile without the immediate response of more highly trained emergency personnel.

## Rapid Activation of EMS

The next link involves the EMS dispatcher who receives the call for help from someone already on the scene. The dispatcher quickly determines what help is needed and sends the appropriate professionals.

## First Responder Care

The first person to arrive on the scene who is trained to provide a higher level of care is often referred to as the **first responder.** This person has the skills to better assess the victim's condition and take appropriate actions, which include caring for life-threatening conditions. First responders have traditionally been police officers and fire fighters. Besides these traditional first responders, others routinely summoned include industrial safety personnel, athletic trainers, and those with similar responsibilities for the safety and well-being of

# Hundreds of Millions Served

In case of emergency, call 9-1-1. Across our country, 9-1-1 service has helped millions of people. You read a news article about a 5-year-old boy who saves his 8-year-old brother or an infant who is saved by his mother. They were instructed in lifesaving first aid over the phone by the 9-1-1 emergency dispatcher. Why 9-1-1? Why does it exist?

The 9-1-1 service was created in the United States in 1968 as a nationwide telephone number for the public to use to report emergencies and request emergency assistance. It gives the public direct access to a Public Service Answering Point that is responsible for taking the appropriate action. The numbers 9-1-1 were chosen because they best fit the needs of the public and the telephone company. They are easy to remember and dial, and they have never been used as an office, area, or service code.[1]

When should you call 9-1-1? Call 9-1-1 whenever there is a threat to life or property, or the potential for injury.[2] Fire and motor vehicle crashes are obvious emergencies that require using 9-1-1. But you should also call 9-1-1 for other situations that threaten life or property, or those that may cause injury such as a dangerous animal running loose, a downed electrical line, a burglary, or an assault.

Hundreds of millions of people call 9-1-1 each year. The majority, approximately 80 percent of 9-1-1 calls, pertain to law enforcement. Fire and EMS comprise the rest. EMS professionals alone respond to more than 19 million 9-1-1 calls each year.

What advantages does 9-1-1 offer? It was designed to save time in the overall response of a public safety agency (for example, fire, police, EMS) to a call for help.[1] This includes the time it takes a citizen to telephone the correct agency or agencies for help. For example, imagine that a house is on fire in your neighborhood and your neighbor has been seriously burned. You run to call for help. Whom should you call first—the fire department to come and put out the fire so no one else is hurt, the ambulance so EMTs can attend to your neighbor, or the police

to help secure the area? Without 9-1-1 service, you may need to place separate calls to all three agencies.

With 9-1-1 service, regardless of your needs, you make only one call. When the call comes in, a 9-1-1 dispatcher answers the call, listens to the caller, gathers needed information, and dispatches help.

Perhaps one of the most exciting lifesaving advances in computer technology in the past few years has been the development of an enhanced 9-1-1 system.

This system uses Computer-Aided Dispatch (CAD). As soon as a call comes in, CAD automatically displays the telephone number, address, and name in which the phone is listed. So, even if the caller is unable to remain on the line or unable to speak or if the call is disconnected, the dispatcher has enough information to send help.

The latest advance in 9-1-1 system development is the use of CAD units in police cars, fire engines, and ambulances. By the time personnel start these vehicles, the built-in CAD units provide them with the location information. These CAD units are also used to send messages, establishing a vital communication link among the caller, the dispatcher, and the field unit en route.

With all of its advantages and lifesaving capabilities, 9-1-1 service today covers only approximately 50 percent of the U.S. population. While 125 cities with over 100,000 people have 9-1-1 service, other areas of the country are still without this lifesaving service.[2] As more cities establish 9-1-1 systems, response times of emergency personnel will continue to improve resulting in more lives being saved.

**REFERENCES**

1. National Emergency Number Association: *Nine one one 9-1-1 (what's it all about?)*.
2. Stanton W, Executive Director, National Emergency Number Association: Interview, Feb 13, 1990.

others. Because of the nature of their job, first responders are often close to the scene and frequently have appropriate supplies and equipment. Their care often provides a critical transition between a citizen's initial actions and the care of more highly trained professionals.

## More Advanced Prehospital Care

The arrival of **emergency medical technicians (EMTs)** represents the next link in the chain of survival (Fig. 1-2). Depending on the level of training and certification (basic, intermediate, or paramedic), the EMT can provide more advanced care and life-support techniques. An EMT's training requires successful completion of a state-approved EMT training program, which provides experience in both prehospital and hospital settings. In most parts of the United States, ambulance personnel must be certified at least at the basic EMT level.

**Paramedics** (EMT-Ps) are highly specialized EMTs. In addition to performing basic EMT skills, paramedics can administer medication and intravenous fluids and deliver advanced care for breathing problems and abnormal heart rhythms. Paramedics provide the highest level of prehospital care. They serve as the field extension of the emergency physician. Regardless of the level of training, the EMT's role is to reassess the victim's condition and to begin and continue appropriate care until the victim reaches the hospital.

## Hospital Care

When the victim arrives at the hospital emergency department, the emergency department staff takes over care (Fig. 1-3). Many personnel in this link become involved as needed, including physicians, nurses, and other health care professionals.

A nurse trained to assess the victim's condition is usually the first member of the emergency department staff involved. He or she quickly evaluates the victim and identifies any immediate threats to the victim's life. Other specially trained emergency department nurses continue to provide needed care.

Most hospital emergency departments are staffed by emergency department physicians, trained to care for the acutely ill or injured. They provide care that further stabilizes a critically ill or injured person. If more specialized care is required, the emergency department physician involves the appropriate medical

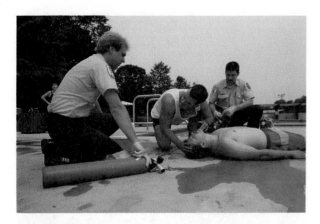

**Figure 1-2**   EMTs often take over for first responders and provide a higher level of care.

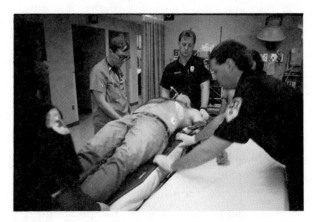

**Figure 1-3**   At the hospital, EMTs turn over care of the victim to the emergency department staff.

specialist: for example, a cardiologist, orthopedic surgeon, neurosurgeon, or trauma surgeon.

In addition to nurses and physicians, many other allied health personnel may help provide care. These include respiratory technicians, radiology technicians, and laboratory technicians.

## Rehabilitation

The final link in the chain of survival is **rehabilitation.** The goal of rehabilitation is to return the victim to his or her previous state of health. This phase begins once the medical problem has been corrected. Other health care professionals, including family physicians, consulting specialists, social workers, and physical therapists, work together to rehabilitate the victim.

## ◆ SUPPORTING THE EMS SYSTEM

The chain of survival depends on all people in the chain performing their roles correctly and promptly to make the EMS system work. Citizens must (1) recognize emergencies and quickly enlist help by activating the system, (2) learn which actions to take in the first critical minutes, and (3) learn to prevent emergencies and be prepared for them. They need to support the EMS system in their community.

Professional rescuers must respond sensitively, quickly, and effectively to emergencies when they are summoned. They must keep their training current and stay abreast of new issues in emergency response. Each link in the chain working effectively enhances the victim's chances for a full recovery.

What happens if one of the links in the chain of survival breaks? Since the victim's life may depend on each or all of these links, a broken link can cause serious consequences.

For instance, if a citizen responder does not recognize a life-threatening emergency, such as the early signals of a heart attack, and does not quickly call EMS personnel, the victim may not live. Poor information given to the EMS dispatcher may delay advanced care. Improper care of the victim before more advanced care arrives can result in the condition worsening.

In a serious injury or illness, survival and recovery are not a matter of chance. Survival results from a carefully orchestrated chain of events in which all participants fulfill their roles. The EMS system can make the difference between life and death or a partial or full recovery. *You,* as a professional rescuer, play a critical role in this system.

## ◆ LEGAL CONSIDERATIONS

Many people are concerned about lawsuits. Lawsuits against those who give care at the scene of an emergency, however, are highly unusual and rarely successful. By being aware of some basic legal principles, you may be able to avoid any possible legal action in the future (Fig. 1-4).

The following sections address in general terms the legal principles that concern emer-

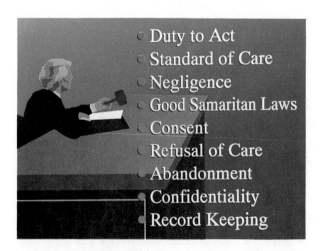

- Duty to Act
- Standard of Care
- Negligence
- Good Samaritan Laws
- Consent
- Refusal of Care
- Abandonment
- Confidentiality
- Record Keeping

**Figure 1-4**  Professional rescuers should be aware of basic legal considerations.

gency care. Because laws vary from state to state, you should inquire about specific laws in your state.

## Duty to Act

Most professional rescuers, either by **case law, statute,** or job description, have a **duty to act** at the scene of an emergency. This duty applies to public safety officers, government employees, licensed and certified professionals, and paraprofessionals while on duty. For instance, members of a volunteer fire department have a duty to act based on their agreement to participate in the fire department. An athletic trainer has a duty to give care to an injured athlete. An EMT, nurse, or physician has a duty to provide care to a patient. Failure to adhere to these agreements could result in legal action.

## Standard of Care

The public expects a certain **standard of care** from personnel summoned to provide emergency care. For example, the standard of care for first responders and EMTs is based on the training guidelines developed by the U.S. Department of Transportation and by the states and municipalities in which they serve. State laws and other authorities, such as national organizations, may govern the actions of other professional rescuers. If your actions do not meet the standards set for you, you may be successfully sued if your actions harm another person.

## Negligence

**Negligence** is the failure to follow a reasonable standard of care, thereby causing injury or damage to another. A person could be negligent either by acting wrongly or failing to act at all. For example, ignoring or misinterpreting signals of a heart attack, failing to give the victim appropriate care, or not summoning more advanced life support personnel could be construed as negligence.

## Good Samaritan Laws

Most states have enacted **Good Samaritan laws,** which protect people providing emergency care. These laws will generally protect you from legal liability as long as you act in good faith, are not negligent, act within the scope of your training, and do not accept anything in return for your services. Since Good Samaritan laws differ from state to state, you should check with a lawyer in your area to determine the extent to which these laws protect you.

## Consent

A person has the basic right to decide what can and cannot be done with his or her body. Therefore, before you can provide care, you must first obtain that person's **consent.**

To obtain consent, you must—
1. Identify yourself to the person.
2. Give your level of training.
3. Explain what you think may be wrong.
4. Explain what you plan to do.

After you have provided this information, the person can decide whether to grant his or her **informed consent.** A person can withdraw consent at any time.

Unless a life-threatening condition exists, a parent or adult guardian who is present must grant consent for a minor before care can be given. You may encounter a situation in which a parent or guardian refuses to allow you to give needed care. In such cases, law enforcement personnel can help to obtain the necessary legal authority to provide care. This also holds true for adults who are under a legal guardian's care.

A person who is unconscious, confused, or seriously ill may not be able to grant consent. In such cases the law assumes the person would grant consent if able to do so. This is termed **"implied consent."** Implied consent also applies to minors who obviously need emergency assistance when a parent or guardian is not present.

## Refusal of Care

Some ill or injured people, even those who desperately need care, may refuse the care you offer. Even though the person may have a serious condition, you should honor his or her **refusal of care.** Try to convince the person of the need for care, but do not argue. Allow more advanced medical personnel to evaluate

the situation. If possible, to make it clear that you did not abandon the person, have a witness hear the person's refusal, and document it. Many EMS systems have a "Refusal of Care" form that can be used in these situations.

## Abandonment

Just as you must have consent from a person before beginning care, you must also continue to give care once you have begun. Once you have started emergency care, you are legally obligated to continue that care until a person with equal or higher training relieves you. Usually, your obligation for care ends when

## The Right to Choose

You respond to a call dispatched as a "Heart Attack." A woman has advised that her husband was found unconscious and not breathing. Once on the scene, you ask how long he has been like this. The woman responds, "I don't know." You check a 60-year-old man for vital signs. No pulse! You are suddenly faced with the fact that the victim is clinically dead.

You've been trained to start CPR when there is no pulse. But the victim's wife tells you *not* to resuscitate him. She shows you papers that state his wishes not to receive medical care. Questions race through your mind. What are my moral and legal responsibilities? Is this document valid? Should I start CPR anyway? Should I call for advice? Should I follow my local protocols? Do my protocols cover this situation?

According to the Journal of the American Medical Association (JAMA), "When a person suffers a cardiac arrest, prompt initiation of CPR is indicated. CPR should be provided by trained personnel unless generally accepted criteria for the determination of death are met or there is documentation of other reliable reasons to believe that CPR is not indicated, wanted, or in the victim's best interest."

Written instructions that describe a person's wishes about medical treatment are called *ad-*

*vance directives.* These instructions are used when the person can no longer make his or her own health care decisions.

Some examples of advance directives are *living wills* and *durable powers of attorney for health care.* The types of health care decisions covered by these documents vary depending on where you live. Talking with a legal professional can help determine which advance directive options are available in your state and what they do and do not cover.

Living wills generally allow a person to refuse only medical care that "merely prolongs the process of dying."

A durable power of attorney for health care is a document authorizing someone to make medical decisions for an individual if that individual should become unable to make them for him or herself. This authorized person should support the needs and wishes of the victim, as outlined in the advance directive.

Another way to formalize preferences is by using *Do Not Resuscitate (DNR)* orders. A doctor could make DNR orders a part of an individual's medical record. Such orders would state that if the individual's heartbeat or breathing stops, he or she should not be resuscitated. The choice in deciding on DNR orders may be cov-

more advanced medical professionals take over. If you stop your care before that point, you can be legally responsible for the **abandonment** of a person in need.

## Confidentiality

While providing care, you may learn things about the victim that are generally considered private and confidential. Information such as previous medical problems, physical problems, and medications being taken is personal to the victim. Respect the victim's privacy by maintaining **confidentiality.** Television and newspaper reporters may ask you questions.

Attorneys may also approach you at the scene. Never discuss the victim or the care you gave with anyone except law enforcement personnel or other personnel caring for the victim.

## Record Keeping

Documenting your care is nearly as important as the care itself. Because a victim's condition may change, a record of the condition immediately after the emergency will provide useful information. Others providing care can compare the current condition to what you recorded earlier.

Your record is a legal document and is im-

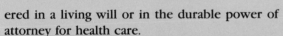

ered in a living will or in the durable power of attorney for health care.

Since these documents are sometimes still unclear about the exact level of care desired, a more recent approach has been to consider establishing *no-CPR* orders to avoid confusion. EMS personnel are encouraged to become familiar with the intent of the order and make provisions to identify persons who have no-CPR orders.

Interpreting advance directives in the prehospital setting is fraught with difficulty; it requires the rescuer to interpret a legal document at the time of a medical emergency. So what is being done to make this decision easier?

EMS systems are developing protocols so that if confronted with an advance directive, the responder will know what to do. In some cases, first responders, EMTs, and paramedics initiate care, but quickly notify their Medical Control Physician of the situation. Since family members may be concerned that emergency medical personnel are not honoring the requests of the advance directive, personnel must sensitively and emphatically convey to the family their responsibility to initiate care while awaiting physician direction.

According to JAMA, "In certain cases, it may

be difficult to determine if resuscitation should be started. For example, despite the presence of a no-CPR order, family members, surrogates, or the patient's physician may request that CPR be initiated. If there is reasonable doubt or substantive reason to believe the no-CPR order is invalid, CPR should be initiated. If evidence later indicates that resuscitation is inappropriate, CPR or other life support can be discontinued."

Advance directives are not limited to elderly people or people with a terminal illness. More people of all ages are choosing to make their wishes known through advance directives.

Prepare yourself for emergency situations by knowing how to handle advance directives. Check with your local EMS system. Inquire about how to deal with living wills, medical durable powers of attorney for health care, DNR orders, and no-CPR orders.

**REFERENCES**

1. Hospital Shared Services of Colorado, Stockard Inventory Program: *Your right to make health care decisions,* Denver, Colo, 1992.
2. Title 42 United States Code, Sections 1395 cc (a) (1) (Q) (A) *Patient Self-Determination Act.*
3. Guidelines for cardiopulmonary resuscitation and emergency cardiac care: recommendations of the 1992 National Conference, *JAMA:* 1992.

portant if legal action occurs. Should you be called to court for any reason, your record will support what you saw, heard, and did at the scene of the emergency. It is important to write the record as soon as possible while all the facts are fresh in your memory (Fig. 1-5). Many systems have printed forms used for record keeping.

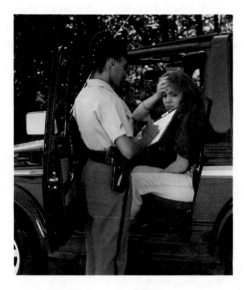

**Figure 1-5**   Record the initial condition of the victim.

## ◆ SUMMARY

The survival and recovery of a seriously ill or injured person depends on all parts of the EMS system working together efficiently. Citizen response, rapid EMS response, first responder care, advanced prehospital care, hospital care, and rehabilitation are the links in the chain of survival.

In your role as an emergency care provider, you are guided by certain legal parameters such as the duty to act and professional standards of care. Effective record keeping is important in maintaining the standard of care and provides legal protection for you and the organization you represent.

## ◆ Review Questions ◆

**1.** Laws that protect people who willingly give emergency care without accepting anything in return are called—
a. Citizen Responder laws.
b. Hold Harmless laws.
c. Good Samaritan laws.
d. Medical Immunity laws.

**2.** Which of the following is a personal characteristic shared by professional rescuers?
a. Controlling all other professional rescuers at an emergency scene
b. Having a duty when on the job to re-

spond in an emergency and provide medical care to the ill and injured
c. Presenting a professional appearance
d. Being trained to provide care at a paramedic level

**3.** Which of the following is a responsibility of professional rescuers?
a. Ensuring personal safety and safety of others
b. Determining any threats to the victim's life
c. Providing needed care for the victim
d. All of the above

**4.** Which statement best describes the emergency medical services system?

a. The EMS system is organized to prevent the occurrence of injuries and sudden illnesses.

b. The EMS system consists of community resources organized to care for victims of sudden illness and injury.

c. The EMS system provides an ambulance to transport victims to the hospital.

d. Personnel and equipment for removing victims from dangerous locations are part of the EMS system.

**5.** Record keeping is important because—

a. The victim may need to read the record when he or she recovers.

b. The hospital emergency department always requires you to present a record.

c. A record gives useful information for those who provide advanced care.

d. A record will be of use to you in another emergency situation.

**6.** To provide care for an ill or injured person, you must first—

a. Acquire that person's consent.

b. Begin to write your record of what happened.

c. Ask bystanders what happened.

d. Find out if you have a duty to act.

Answers: 1. c; 2. c; 3. d; 4. b; 5. c; 6. a

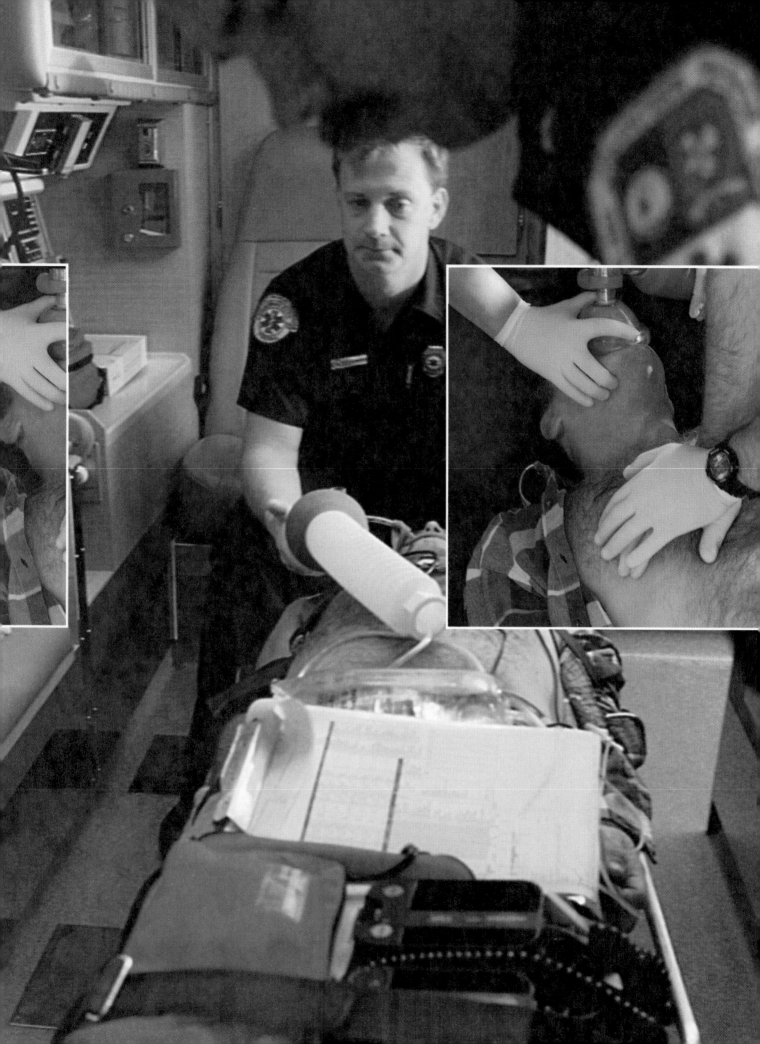

# Part Two

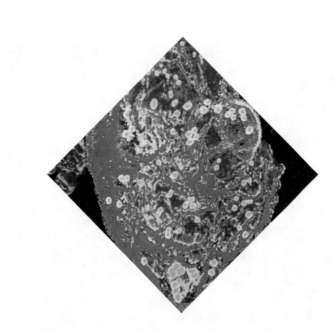

# Understanding the Human Body

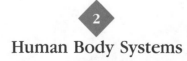

2

Human Body Systems

3

Preventing Disease Transmission

# Human Body Systems

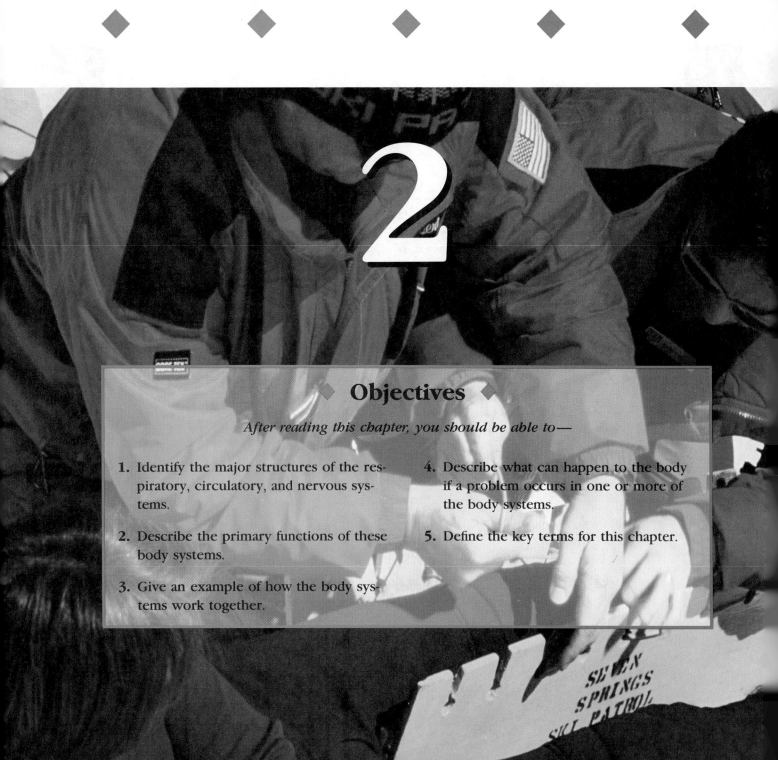

2

## Objectives

*After reading this chapter, you should be able to—*

1. Identify the major structures of the respiratory, circulatory, and nervous systems.

2. Describe the primary functions of these body systems.

3. Give an example of how the body systems work together.

4. Describe what can happen to the body if a problem occurs in one or more of the body systems.

5. Define the key terms for this chapter.

# ◆ Key Terms ◆

**Body systems:** A group of organs and other structures working together to carry out specific functions.

**Cells:** The basic units of all living tissue.

**Circulatory system:** A group of organs and other structures that carries oxygen-rich blood and other nutrients throughout the body and removes waste.

**Nervous system:** A group of organs and other structures that regulates all body functions.

**Organ:** A collection of similar tissues acting together to perform specific body functions.

**Respiratory system:** A group of organs and other structures that brings air into the body and removes wastes through a process called breathing, or respiration.

**Tissue:** A collection of similar cells acting together to perform specific body functions.

**Vital organs:** Organs whose functions are essential to life, including the brain, heart, and lungs.

# ◆ Main Ideas ◆

1. The body needs a constant supply of oxygen for survival.

2. The respiratory and circulatory systems work together to supply oxygen to the brain and the rest of the body.

3. Knowledge of how the respiratory and circulatory systems work can help the professional rescuer perform cardiopulmonary resuscitation (CPR).

## ◆ BODY SYSTEMS

The human body is a miraculous machine. It performs many complex functions, each of which helps us live. The body is composed of billions of microscopic **cells,** the basic unit of all living tissue. Many different types of cells exist; each type contributes in a specific way to keep the body functioning normally. Collections of similar cells form **tissues,** which form **organs** (Fig. 2-1). **Vital organs** are organs whose functions are essential for life and include the brain, heart, and lungs.

A **body system** is a group of organs and other structures especially adapted to perform specific body functions. They work together to carry out a function needed for life. For ex-

ample, the heart, blood, and blood vessels make up the **circulatory system,** which keeps all parts of the body supplied with oxygen-rich blood.

For the body to work properly, all its systems must work well together. As a professional rescuer, you need a basic understanding of important body systems. Knowing how the body normally functions will help you more easily recognize and understand serious illness such as a heart attack. Body systems do not function independently. Each system depends on other systems to function properly. When your body is healthy, your body systems are working well together. However, serious illness will often affect the way several body systems function.

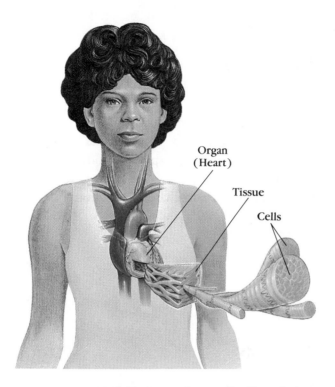

**Figure 2-1**  Organs are made up of cells and tissues.

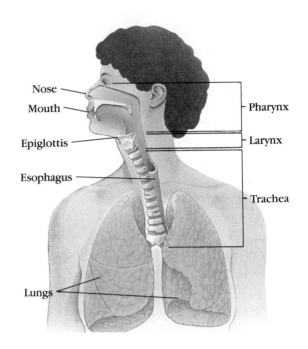

**Figure 2-2**  The Respiratory System

## Respiratory System

### Structure and Function

The body must have a constant supply of oxygen to stay alive. The **respiratory system** supplies the body with oxygen through breathing. When you **inhale,** air fills the lungs and the **oxygen** in the air is transferred to the blood. The blood carries oxygen to all parts of the body. This same system removes **carbon dioxide** when you **exhale,** or breathe out. This breathing process is called **respiration.**

The respiratory system includes the airway and lungs. The **airway,** the passage for air to travel to the lungs, begins at the nose and mouth, which form the upper airway. Air passes through this upper airway, through the **pharynx** (the throat), the **larynx** (the voice box), and the trachea on its way to the lungs (Fig. 2-2). The **lungs** are a pair of organs in the chest that provide the mechanism for taking in oxygen and removing carbon dioxide

during breathing. The **trachea** is also called the windpipe. Behind the trachea is the esophagus. The **esophagus** carries food and liquids from the mouth to the stomach. A small flap of tissue, the **epiglottis,** covers the trachea when a person swallows to keep food and liquids out of the lungs.

Air reaches the lungs through two tubes called **bronchi.** The bronchi branch into increasingly smaller tubes (Fig. 2-3, *A*). These eventually end in millions of tiny air sacs called **alveoli** (Fig. 2-3, *B*). Oxygen and carbon dioxide pass into and out of the blood through the thin cell walls of the alveoli and tiny blood vessels called **capillaries.**

Air enters the lungs when you inhale and leaves the lungs when you exhale. When you inhale, the chest muscles and the **diaphragm** contract. This expands the chest and draws air into the lungs. When you exhale, the chest muscles and diaphragm relax, allowing air to exit from the lungs (Fig. 2-4). The average

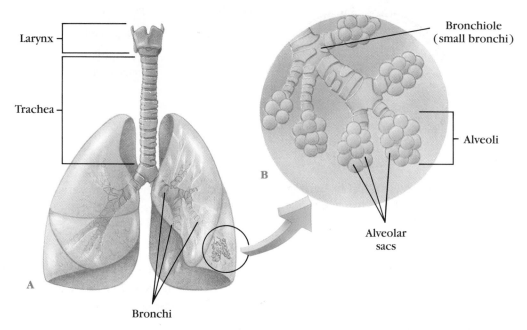

**Figure 2-3** **A,** The bronchi branch into many small tubes. **B,** Oxygen and carbon dioxide pass into and out of blood through the walls of the alveoli and the capillaries.

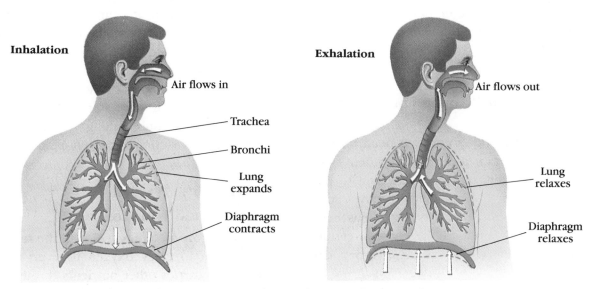

**Figure 2-4** The chest muscles and the diaphragm contract as you inhale and relax as you exhale.

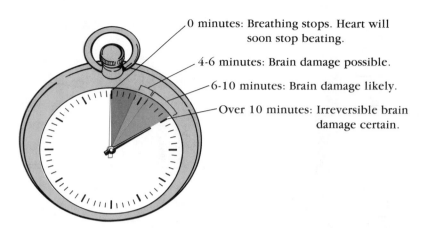

0 minutes: Breathing stops. Heart will soon stop beating.

4-6 minutes: Brain damage possible.

6-10 minutes: Brain damage likely.

Over 10 minutes: Irreversible brain damage certain.

**Figure 2-5**　Time is critical in starting lifesaving measures. If the brain is without oxygen for 6 minutes, brain damage is likely to occur.

adult breathes about one pint of air (500 ml) per breath and about 10 to 20 times per minute.

This ongoing breathing process is involuntary and is controlled by the brain. The brain is the control center for breathing. It adjusts the rate and depth of breaths according to the oxygen and carbon dioxide levels in the body. The brain is very sensitive to oxygen starvation. Without oxygen, brain cells begin to die in as few as 4 to 6 minutes (Fig. 2-5). Other vital organs will also be affected unless oxygen supplies are restored.

## Problems That Require Emergency Care

Because of the body's constant need for oxygen, it is important to recognize when a person is having difficulty breathing and to provide emergency care immediately. Some causes of breathing difficulty include **asthma,** allergies, and injuries to the chest. Breathing difficulty is referred to as **respiratory distress.**

If a person is in respiratory distress, you may hear or see noisy breathing or gasping. The victim may be conscious or unconscious. The conscious victim may be anxious or excited or may say that he or she feels short of breath. The victim's skin, particularly the lips

and under the nails, may have a blue tint. This discoloration is called **cyanosis** and occurs when the tissues do not receive enough oxygen.

If a person stops breathing, it is called **respiratory arrest.** Respiratory arrest is a life-threatening emergency. Without the oxygen obtained from breathing, other body systems fail to function. For example, if the brain does not receive oxygen, it cannot send messages to the heart to beat. The heart will therefore soon stop.

Respiratory problems require immediate attention. Making sure the airway is open and clear is an important first step. You may have to breathe for a nonbreathing victim or clear the airway of a victim who is choking.

## Circulatory System

### Structure and Function

The circulatory system works with the respiratory system to carry oxygen to every body cell. It also carries other nutrients throughout the body and removes waste. The circulatory system includes the heart, blood, and blood vessels (Fig. 2-6).

The **heart** is a muscular organ that circulates blood throughout the body through veins and arteries. **Arteries** are large blood

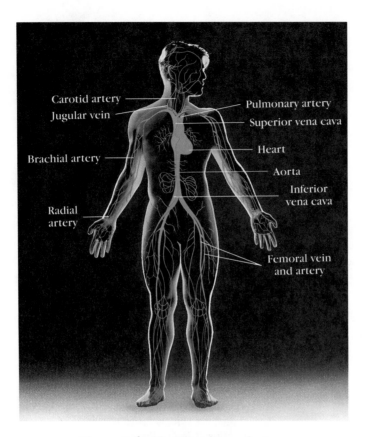

Carotid artery
Jugular vein

Pulmonary artery
Superior vena cava

Brachial artery

Heart

Aorta

Inferior
vena cava

Radial
artery

Femoral vein
and artery

**Figure 2-6** The Circulatory System

vessels that carry oxygen-rich blood from the heart to the rest of the body. The arteries subdivide into smaller blood vessels and ultimately become tiny capillaries. The **capillaries** transport blood to all the cells of the body and nourish them with oxygen.

The heart lies between the lungs, in the middle of the chest, behind the lower half of the **sternum** (breastbone). The heart is protected by the **ribs** and sternum in front and by the spine in back. It has four chambers and is separated into right and left halves. Oxygen-poor blood enters the right side of the heart and is circulated to the lungs, where it picks up oxygen. This oxygen-enriched blood returns to the left side of the heart, where it is circulated to all parts of the body. One-way valves direct the flow of blood as it moves through each of the heart's four chambers (Fig. 2-7). For the circulatory system to be effective, the respiratory system must also

be working so that the blood can pick up oxygen in the lungs and take it to the body cells.

After the oxygen in the blood is given to the cells, **veins** carry the oxygen-poor blood back to the heart. The heart circulates this oxygen-poor blood to the lungs to pick up more oxygen before circulating it to other parts of the body. This cycle is called the **circulatory cycle.**

The beating action of the heart is called a **contraction.** Contractions are controlled by the heart's electrical system, which makes the heart beat regularly. You can feel the heart's contractions in the arteries that are close to the skin, for instance, at the neck or the wrist. The beat you feel with each contraction is called the **pulse.** The heart must beat regularly to deliver oxygen to the body cells to keep the body functioning properly.

Like all living tissue, the cells of the heart

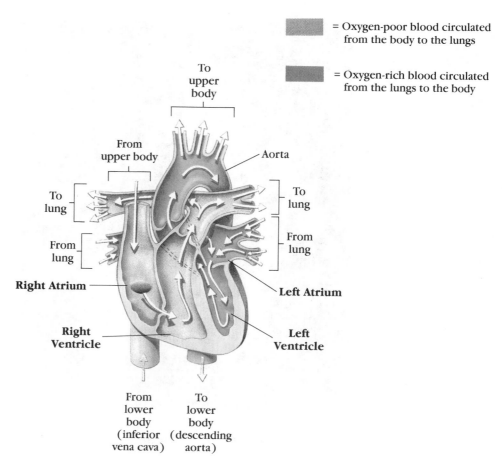

= Oxygen-poor blood circulated from the body to the lungs

= Oxygen-rich blood circulated from the lungs to the body

To upper body

From upper body

Aorta

To lung

To lung

From lung

From lung

**Right Atrium**

**Left Atrium**

**Right Ventricle**

**Left Ventricle**

From lower body (inferior vena cava)

To lower body (descending aorta)

**Figure 2-7** The heart is made up of four chambers. A system of one-way valves keeps blood moving in the proper direction to complete the circulatory cycle.

need a continuous supply of oxygen. The **coronary arteries** supply the heart muscle with oxygen-rich blood.

### Problems That Require Emergency Care

The following problems threaten the delivery of oxygen to the body cells:

- Failure of the heart to circulate blood adequately (example: a heart attack)
- Blood loss caused by severe bleeding (example: a severed artery)
- Impaired circulation (example: a blood clot)

Body tissues that do not receive oxygen die.

For example, when an artery supplying the brain with blood is blocked, brain tissue dies. When an artery supplying the heart with blood is blocked, heart muscle tissue dies. This situation results in a life-threatening emergency such as a heart attack.

If heart muscle tissue is deprived of oxygen-rich blood, it dies. If too much tissue dies, the heart cannot circulate blood effectively; this illness is often called a **heart attack.** A heart attack interrupts the heart's electrical system. This may result in an irregular heartbeat, which prevents blood from circulating effectively. The heart may stop beating. If it does stop, breathing will also stop. When the heart

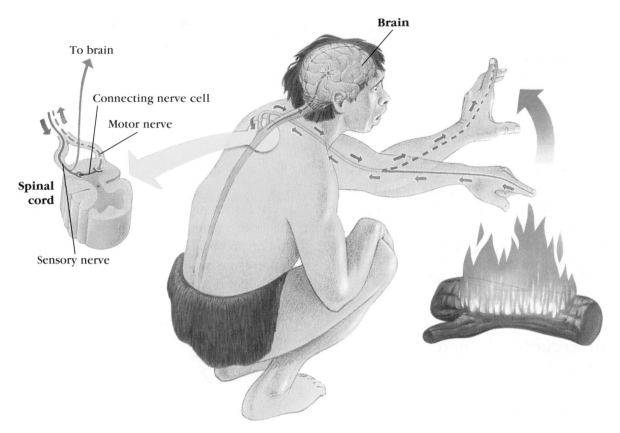

**Figure 2-8** Messages are sent to and from the brain by way of the nerves.

stops or beats too irregularly to circulate blood, the condition is called **cardiac arrest.** Victims of either heart attack or cardiac arrest need emergency care immediately.

Cardiac arrest victims need to have circulation maintained artificially. This is done by both compressing the chest and breathing for the victim. This combination of compressions and breaths is called **cardiopulmonary resuscitation (CPR).**

## Nervous System

### Structure and Function

The **nervous system** is the most complex and delicate of all body systems. The **brain,** the center of the nervous system, is the master organ of the body. It regulates all body functions, including the respiratory and circulatory systems.

The brain transmits and receives information through a network of nerves. The **spinal cord,** a large bundle of nerves, extends from the brain through a canal in the **spine,** or backbone. **Nerves** extend from the brain and spinal cord to every part of the body.

Nerves transmit information as electrical impulses from one area of the body to another. Some nerves conduct impulses from the body to the brain, allowing you to see, hear, smell, taste, and feel. Other nerves conduct impulses from the brain to the muscles to control motor functions, or movement (Fig. 2-8).

The integrated functions of the brain are complex. One of these functions is **consciousness.** Normally, when people are awake, they are conscious. In most cases, being conscious means that you know who you are, where you are, the approximate date and time, and what is happening around you. Various degrees of consciousness exist. A person's **level of consciousness (LOC)** can vary from being highly aware in certain situations to being less aware during periods of relaxation, sleep, illness, or injury.

### Problems That Require Emergency Care

Brain cells, unlike other body cells, cannot regenerate, or grow back. Once brain cells die or are damaged, they are not replaced. Brain cells will die from lack of oxygen. For example, if a victim is unable to breathe because he or she is choking, the victim will eventually lose consciousness. The cells of the brain will begin to die from lack of oxygen.

## Interrelationships of Body Systems

Body systems work together to help the body maintain a constant healthy state. Body systems do not work independently. The impact of injury or illness is rarely restricted to one body system. For example, if the heart stops beating for any reason, breathing will also stop. If the body is deprived of oxygen, brain cells will begin to die within 4 to 6 minutes.

## ◆ SUMMARY

Several body systems must work together for the body to function properly. The primary body systems are the respiratory, circulatory, and nervous systems. The brain, the center of the nervous system, controls all body functions including those of the other body systems. The heart and lungs work together to supply the body with the oxygen needed to support life. Without these systems functioning properly, death will occur.

## ◆ Review Questions ◆

**1.** Which structure in the airway prevents liquids and solids from entering the lungs?
a. Epiglottis
b. Uvula
c. Trachea
d. Esophagus

**2.** Which of the following could result from breathing difficulty or other problems of the respiratory system?
a. The heart could stop beating.
b. Oxygen might not be delivered to all parts of the body.
c. Brain cells could die.
d. All of the above.

**3.** A blood clot in the brain could cut off all blood flow to brain cells. Which body systems would fail to function?
a. Nervous system
b. Circulatory and respiratory systems
c. Nervous and respiratory systems
d. All body systems

Answers. 1. a; 2. d; 3. d

# Preventing Disease Transmission

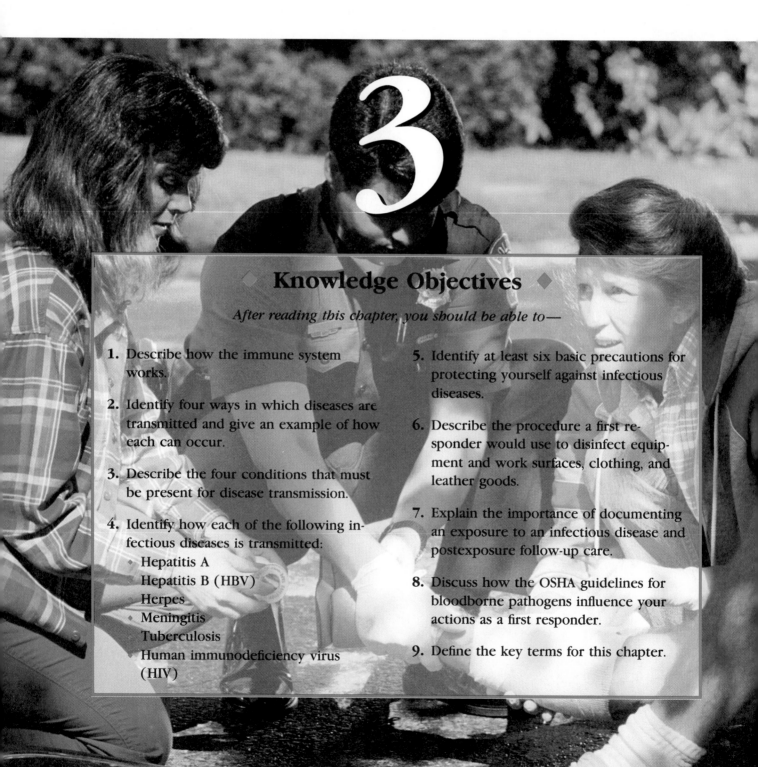

3

## ◆ Knowledge Objectives ◆

*After reading this chapter, you should be able to—*

1. Describe how the immune system works.

2. Identify four ways in which diseases are transmitted and give an example of how each can occur.

3. Describe the four conditions that must be present for disease transmission.

4. Identify how each of the following infectious diseases is transmitted:
   - Hepatitis A
   - Hepatitis B (HBV)
   - Herpes
   - Meningitis
   - Tuberculosis
   - Human immunodeficiency virus (HIV)

5. Identify at least six basic precautions for protecting yourself against infectious diseases.

6. Describe the procedure a first responder would use to disinfect equipment and work surfaces, clothing, and leather goods.

7. Explain the importance of documenting an exposure to an infectious disease and postexposure follow-up care.

8. Discuss how the OSHA guidelines for bloodborne pathogens influence your actions as a first responder.

9. Define the key terms for this chapter.

# ◆ Key Terms ◆

**AIDS (acquired immune deficiency syndrome):** A condition caused by the human immunodeficiency virus (HIV).

**Airborne transmission:** The transmission of a disease by inhaling infected droplets that become airborne when an infected person coughs or sneezes.

**Bacteria (Bac TE re ah):** One-celled microorganisms that may cause infections.

**Bloodborne pathogens:** Bacteria and viruses present in human blood and body fluids that can cause disease in humans.

**Body substance isolation (BSI):** An infection control strategy that considers all body substances as potentially infectious.

**Direct contact transmission:** The transmission of a disease by touching an infected person's body fluids.

**Hepatitis (hep ah TI tis):** A viral infection of the liver.

**Herpes (HER pēz):** A viral infection that causes eruptions of the skin and mucous membranes.

**HIV (human immunodeficiency virus):** The virus that destroys the body's ability to fight infection. The resultant state is referred to as AIDS.

**Immune system:** The body's group of responses for fighting disease.

**Immunization (im u nĭ ZA shun):** A specific substance containing weakened or killed pathogens that is introduced into the body to build resistance to specific infection.

**Indirect contact transmission:** The transmission of a disease by touching a contaminated object.

**Infection:** A condition caused by disease-producing microorganisms, called pathogens or germs, in the body.

**Infectious disease:** Disease capable of being transmitted from people, objects, animals, or insects.

**Meningitis (men in JI tis):** An inflammation of the brain or spinal cord caused by a viral or bacterial infection.

**Pathogen (PATH o jen):** A disease-causing agent; also called a microorganism or germ.

**Tuberculosis (tu ber ku LO sis) (TB):** A respiratory disease caused by a bacterium.

**Universal precautions:** Safety measures taken to prevent occupational-risk exposure to blood or other body fluids containing visible blood.

**Vector transmission:** The transmission of a disease by an animal or insect bite through exposure to blood or other body fluids.

**Virus (VI rus):** A disease-causing agent, or pathogen, that requires another organism to live and reproduce.

# ◆ Main Ideas ◆

1. The Occupational Safety and Health Administration (OSHA) has issued regulations to reduce or remove the hazards of on-the-job exposure to bloodborne pathogens.

2. Herpes, meningitis, tuberculosis, hepatitis, and HIV infection, including AIDS, are infections that can have serious consequences if transmitted.

3. Employers are required to have an Exposure Control Plan to protect employees from infection.

4. In order to prevent disease transmission, you must follow basic precautions each time you prepare to provide care.

## ◆ INTRODUCTION

On December 6, 1991, the Occupational Safety and Health Administration (OSHA) issued final regulations on job exposure to bloodborne pathogens. These are bacteria and viruses present in human blood and other body fluids that can cause disease in humans. OSHA has determined that employees are at risk when they are exposed on the job to blood and other materials that may cause infections. These materials may contain certain **pathogens,** or germs. These pathogens include **hepatitis B** virus (HBV) that causes hepatitis B, a serious liver disease, and **human immunodeficiency virus (HIV),** which causes AIDS.

OSHA has concluded that employers can reduce or remove this hazard from the workplace. This can be done by using a combination of engineering and work practice controls, personal protective clothing and equipment, training, medical surveillance, hepatitis B vaccination, signs and labels, and other provisions.

### Who Is Covered by This Regulation?

The regulation defines the range of employees it covers. It includes any employee for whom there is a "reasonable anticipation" of exposure to blood or other materials that could cause infections, while on the job. The hazard of exposure to infectious materials affects employees in many types of jobs. It extends beyond the health care industry. Employees in the following jobs are covered by this standard if they have on-the-job exposure:

- Employees in health care facilities
- Employees in clinics in factories, schools, and prisons
- Employees assigned to provide emergency first aid
- Employees who handle regulated waste
- Emergency medical technicians, paramedics, and others who provide emergency medical services
- Fire fighters, law enforcement officers, and corrections officers (employees in the pri-

vate sector, the Federal government, or a state or local government in a state that has an OSHA-approved state plan)
- Linen service employees

The standard does *not* cover any "Good Samaritan" actions that result in exposure to blood or other infectious materials.

### Why Take Training?

At some time, you may be concerned about disease transmission. You need to understand how infections occur, how they are passed from one person to another, and what you can do to protect yourself and others.

Diseases that can be contracted from people, objects, animals, or insects are often called infectious diseases. Some diseases can be transmitted more easily than others. You need to know how to recognize situations that have the potential for **disease transmission** and how to protect yourself and others from contracting a disease.

## ◆ HOW INFECTIONS OCCUR
## Disease-Causing Agents

The disease process begins when a pathogen (germ) gets into the body. When pathogens enter the body, they can sometimes overpower the body's defense system and cause illness. This illness is an infection. Most **infectious diseases** are caused by one of the six types of pathogens (Table 3-1). The most common are viruses and bacteria.

**Bacteria** are everywhere (Fig. 3-1). They do not depend on other organisms for life and can live outside the human body. Most bacteria do not infect humans. Those that do may cause serious illness. Meningitis, scarlet fever, and tetanus are examples of disease caused by bacteria. The body has difficulty fighting infections caused by bacteria. Doctors may prescribe medications called **antibiotics** that either kill the bacteria or weaken them enough for the body to get rid of them. Commonly used antibiotics include penicillin, erythromycin, and tetracycline.

Unlike bacteria, **viruses** depend on other

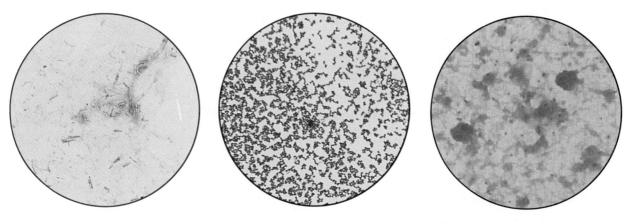

**Figure 3-1** *Mycobacterium tuberculosis, Streptococcus agalactiae,* and *Neisseria meningitidis* are common types of bacteria that cause disease.

| Table 3-1 | Disease-Causing Agents |
| --- | --- |
| **Pathogen** | **Diseases and conditions they cause** |
| Viruses | Hepatitis, measles, mumps, chicken pox, meningitis, rubella, influenza, warts, colds, herpes, shingles, HIV infection including AIDS, genital warts |
| Bacteria | Tetanus, meningitis, scarlet fever, strep throat, tuberculosis, gonorrhea, syphilis, chlamydia, toxic shock syndrome, Legionnaires' disease, diphtheria, food poisoning |
| Fungi | Athlete's foot and ringworm |
| Protozoa | Malaria and dysentery |
| Rickettsia | Typhus, Rocky Mountain spotted fever |
| Parasitic worms | Abdominal pain, anemia, lymphatic vessel blockage, lowered antibody response, respiratory and circulatory complications |

## The Body's Natural Defenses

The body's immune system is very good at fighting disease. Its basic tools are the white blood cells. Special white blood cells travel around the body identifying invading pathogens. Once they detect an invading pathogen, these white blood cells gather around it and release antibodies that fight infections.

These antibodies attack the pathogen and weaken or destroy it. Antibodies usually can get rid of the pathogen. However, once inside the body, some pathogens can thrive and, under ideal conditions, overwhelm the immune system. To minimize this possibility, the body depends on the skin for protection to keep pathogens out.

This combination of trying to keep pathogens out of the body and destroying them

organisms to live and reproduce (Fig. 3-2). Viruses cause many diseases, including the common cold. Once they become established within the body, they are difficult to eliminate because very few medications are effective against them. Antibiotics do not kill or weaken viruses. The body's **immune system** is the main defense against them.

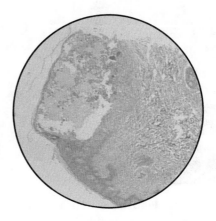

**Figure 3-2** Herpes simplex virus type 2 is a microorganism that causes herpes simplex.

once they get inside is necessary for good health. Sometimes, the body cannot fight off infection. When this occurs, an invading pathogen can become established in the body, causing serious infection. Fever and feeling exhausted often signal that the body is fighting an infection. Other common signals include headache, nausea, and vomiting.

## How Diseases Spread

For a disease to be transmitted, all four of the following conditions must be met:

♦ A pathogen is present.
♦ There is enough of the pathogen to cause disease.
♦ A person is susceptible to the pathogen.
♦ The pathogen passes through the correct entry site.

You need to understand these four conditions to understand how infections occur. Think of these conditions as the pieces of a puzzle. All the pieces have to be in place for the picture to be complete (Fig. 3-3). If any one of these conditions is missing, an infection cannot occur.

Pathogens enter the body in four ways (Fig. 3-4, *A-D*):

♦ Direct contact
♦ Indirect contact
♦ Airborne
♦ Vector-borne

Not all pathogens can enter the body in all of these ways. For example, certain infections are vector-borne only.

**Direct contact transmission** occurs when a person touches body fluids from an infected person. **Indirect contact transmission** occurs when a person touches objects that have touched the blood or another body fluid, such as vomit or saliva, of an infected person. These include soiled dressings, equipment, and work surfaces with which an infected person comes in contact. Sharp objects present a particular risk. If sharp objects have contacted the blood or other body fluids of an infected person and are handled carelessly, they can pierce the skin and transmit infection.

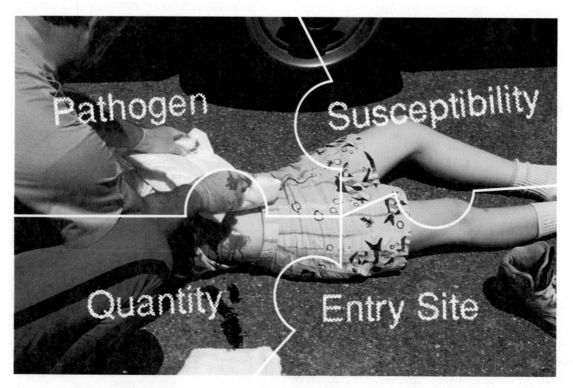

**Figure 3-3** For an infection to occur, all four conditions must be present.

**Airborne transmission** occurs when a person breathes in droplets that become airborne when an infected person coughs or sneezes. If a person is coughing heavily, avoid face-to-face contact, if possible.

**Vector transmission** occurs when an animal, such as a dog or raccoon, or an insect, such as a tick, transmits a pathogen into the body through a bite. A bite from an infected human also is a vector-borne transmission. The carrier is a vector and passes the infection to another animal or person. Rabies and Lyme disease are transmitted this way. You are not usually at risk for vector-borne transmission while on the job.

### ◆ DISEASES THAT CAUSE CONCERN

Some diseases, such as the common cold, are passed from one person to another more easily than others. Although it causes discomfort, the common cold is short-lived and rarely causes serious problems. Other diseases cause more severe problems (Table 3-2). Hepatitis B, a liver infection, can last many months. The patient is often seriously ill and slow to recover. Another infection, caused by the human immunodeficiency virus (HIV), destroys the body's ability to fight infection. Both infections can cause prolonged illness or death.

You should be familiar with diseases that can have severe consequences if transmitted. These include herpes, meningitis, tuberculosis, hepatitis, and HIV infection, the virus that causes AIDS.

### Herpes

Several viruses can cause **herpes** infections. These viruses cause infections of the skin and mucous membranes. They are very easily

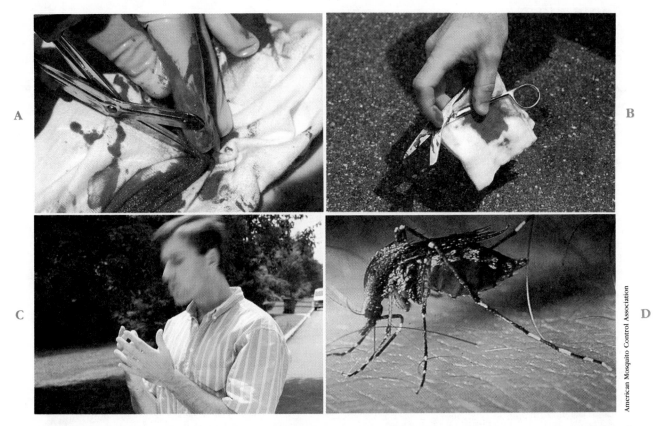

**Figure 3-4** **A,** Direct contact transmission, **B,** indirect contact transmission, **C,** airborne transmission, and **D,** vector transmission are the four ways pathogens can enter the body.

passed by direct contact. The herpes virus stays inactive until stimulated. The early stages of herpes may cause headache, sore throat, swelling of the lymph glands, and a general ill feeling. Sometimes swelling occurs around the lips and mouth where small sores like blisters may form (Fig. 3-5). These are commonly called *cold sores.*

In a more serious form of herpes, sores appear on the face, neck, and shoulders. Another form of herpes causes sores in the genital area. Since antibiotics do not work against viruses, the infection runs its course and becomes inactive for a while. It then flares up again. Herpes is usually transmitted through direct contact with sores. It enters through an opening in the skin or through mucous membranes, such as in the mouth or eyes. You should avoid unprotected contact with people who have active herpes.

## Meningitis

**Meningitis** is a severe infection of the covering of the brain and spinal cord. It can be caused by either viruses or bacteria. It is easily transmitted by direct, indirect, and airborne means.

A person can get the viral form of meningitis from contaminated food and water. Bacterial meningitis can be transmitted through the mucus in the nose and mouth. The germs might be passed if an infected person coughs near another's face or if someone comes in direct contact with the infected person's mucus. You could get bacterial meningitis from unprotected rescue breathing.

Although meningitis is more common in infants and young children, adults are not immune. The first signals are often respiratory infections, sore throat, stiff neck, rash, nausea, and vomiting. An infected person may quickly become seriously ill. In its advanced stages, a person may become unconscious. Meningitis, if treated early, is rarely fatal.

## Tuberculosis

**Tuberculosis** most often affects the respiratory system. The bacteria that cause it live in the lungs. Infection occurs mainly from inhal-

### Table 3-2  How Diseases Are Transmitted

| Disease | Signs and symptoms | Mode of transmission | Infective material |
|---|---|---|---|
| Herpes | Lesions, general ill feeling, sore throat | Direct contact | Broken skin, mucous membranes |
| Meningitis | Respiratory illness, sore throat, nausea, vomiting | Airborne, direct and indirect contact | Food and water, mucus |
| Tuberculosis | Weight loss, night sweats, occasional fever, general ill feeling | Airborne | Saliva, airborne droplets |
| Hepatitis | Flulike, jaundice | Direct and indirect contact | Blood, saliva, semen, feces, food, water, other products |
| HIV | Fever, night sweats, weight loss, chronic diarrhea, severe fatigue, shortness of breath, swollen lymph nodes, lesions | Direct and indirect contact | Blood, semen, vaginal fluid |

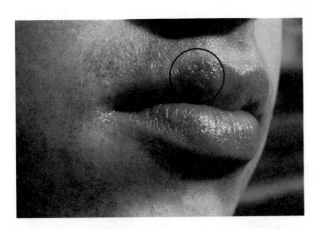

**Figure 3-5** The herpes virus may cause blister-like sores to erupt on or around the lips and mouth.

ing droplets that contain the bacteria. The disease causes weight loss, night sweats, occasional fever, and a general feeling of tiredness. The signals often develop gradually so people may not notice the early stages. People who do not know they have tuberculosis may even remain in fairly good health for a long time before they rapidly become ill.

Recently, a new strain of TB, multiple drug resistant TB (MDR-TB), has been on the rise. This strain commonly results from an infected patient's failure to follow or complete prescribed treatment, resulting in an incomplete destruction of the TB bacteria. The remaining bacteria grow resistant to the antibiotic and subsequently spread to a point that the patient suffers a relapse infection which no longer can be treated with the same medication. Treatment for MDR-TB is based upon timely diagnosis and appropriate administration of medications. MDR-TB may be transmitted as easily as non-resistant TB. Risk of exposure for both strains results from direct contact with respiratory secretions from coughing, spitting, speaking, or singing.

## Hepatitis

Hepatitis is an inflammation of the liver. The most common forms of hepatitis are caused by alcohol abuse, drugs, or other chemicals and cannot be transmitted. Viruses, however, also can cause hepatitis. The two most common types of viral hepatitis are type A and type B.

**Hepatitis A** is also called infectious hepatitis. It is common in children. It is often transmitted by contact with food or other products soiled by the stool of an infected person. Parents may get the disease from their children by changing diapers. Shellfish and water containing the virus also can transmit hepatitis A.

People with hepatitis A at first feel as if they have flu. Later, their skin may become a yellowish color, a condition called jaundice. Hepatitis A usually does not have serious consequences.

Hepatitis B is a severe liver infection caused by the hepatitis B virus. Hepatitis B is primarily transmitted by sexual contact and blood-to-blood contact from transfusions, needle sticks, cuts, scrapes, sores, and skin irritations. Hepatitis B has also been found in other body fluids such as saliva.

Hepatitis B is not transmitted by casual contact, such as shaking hands. It is not transmitted by indirect contact with objects like drinking fountains or telephones. Risk most often occurs in unprotected direct or indirect contact with infected blood.

The signals of hepatitis B are similar to the flulike signals of hepatitis A. Hepatitis B infections can be fatal. The disease may be in the body for up to six months before signals appear. The person may then overlook the flulike signals. Some people can even develop chronic hepatitis after recovering from the early signals.

Non-A−non-B hepatitis is a third form of hepatitis. If a virus cannot be clearly identified as hepatitis A or hepatitis B, it is labeled non-A−non-B. There are several strains of non-A−non-B hepatitis. Recently, one strain has been identified and labeled "hepatitis C." It is believed that hepatitis C is transmitted in the same manner as hepatitis B. The signals present with hepatitis C are similar to those of hepatitis B.

## HIV

**AIDS (acquired immunodeficiency syndrome)** is a result of a weakened immune system. It is caused by HIV (human immunodeficiency virus). This virus attacks white blood cells and destroys the body's ability to fight infection. The infections that strike people whose immune systems are weakened by HIV or other conditions include severe pneumonia and fungal infections of the mouth and esophagus. HIV-infected people may also develop Kaposi's sarcoma and other unusual cancers (Fig. 3-6).

People infected with HIV may not feel or look sick. A blood test, however, can detect the HIV antibody. When the infected person shows signs of having certain infections or cancers, he or she may be diagnosed as having AIDS. The infections can cause severe fatigue, fever, night sweats, unexplained weight loss, chronic diarrhea, shortness of breath, swollen lymph nodes, and skin lesions. In the advanced stages, AIDS is a very serious condition. Victims get life-threatening infections.

It is important to remember the following points about the transmission of HIV:

1. HIV cannot be spread through casual contact.
2. The virus that causes HIV infection is easily killed by alcohol, chlorine bleach, and other common disinfectants. You cannot

# HIV and AIDS

Walter is a businessman in a small town in northern California. He has been a respected member of the community for many years, does volunteer work whenever possible, and is a member of the local Rotary Club. A few years ago, Walter had bypass surgery after a heart attack and was transfused with several pints of blood. As a result of those transfusions, Walter became infected with HIV, the virus that causes AIDS.

Walter is like most of us, has similar dreams, hopes, and fears. He may be a personal friend of yours. Seeing him on the street, you would not guess that he has tested positive for HIV. He will most likely develop AIDS someday and most likely he will die as a result.

Walter is fortunate that he has a supportive network of family and friends. Not everyone is this fortunate. Many suffer because of the irrational fears and rejections of family and friends based on incorrect perceptions.

Human tendency is to protect ourselves against any risks we perceive, correctly or incorrectly. Correct perceptions about HIV and AIDS develop as a result of learning the facts about how HIV is transmitted. Incorrect perceptions involve jumping to conclusions without knowing the facts.

Many people tend to associate the risk of HIV infection with specific groups such as drug users, homosexuals, and members of certain ethnic groups. It is not who a person *is* that puts him or her at risk for HIV infection, but rather what that person *does*. Engaging in unsafe sexual practices or using contaminated intravenous needles are examples of risky behavior that increases the chances of HIV infection.

You will rarely know the details of a person's lifestyle and history when you are giving care in an emergency. Value judgments and jumping to conclusions about someone's behavior play no part in what is required of you. Compassion, understanding, and effective care do. The person you are least likely to suspect may be infected; the one who appears to you to be a more obvious risk may not be. The only physical danger to you occurs when you feel so secure in a situation that you neglect to take the safety precautions that prevent disease transmission. The danger to you as a person exists when you allow preconceptions and prejudices to interfere with those qualities that are an important component of being a first responder.

bring a dead virus back to life by adding water.

3. HIV is known to be transmitted only through exposure to infected blood, semen, vaginal secretions, or (rarely) breast milk. This can occur by—

- Having unprotected sex with an infected partner, male or female.
- Being exposed to blood through use of soiled equipment or supplies, needlestick injuries, or blood splashed on mucous membranes or broken skin. (The risk of getting infected through a blood transfusion or blood product is very low since 1985.)
- Sharing needles or syringes for street drugs, steroids, or ear piercing.
- Being infected as an unborn child or shortly after birth by an infected mother.

> Since 1985, all donated blood in the United States has been tested for HIV antibodies. As a result, the blood supply is considered extremely safe. The risk of becoming infected through a blood transfusion is very low.

## Childhood Diseases

Most people have been immunized against the common childhood diseases such as measles

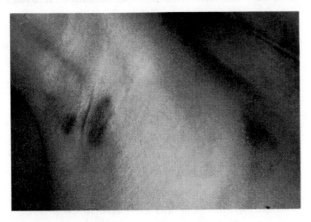

**Figure 3-6**  Kaposi's sarcoma is one of several opportunistic conditions that may strike the HIV-infected person.

and mumps. An **immunization** is the introduction of a substance that contains specific weakened or killed pathogens into the body. The body's immune system then builds a resistance to the specific infection.

No immunization exists, however, for chicken pox (varicella). The varicella infection causes fever and characteristic "pox" (blisterlike sores on the skin). Once you have had chicken pox, it is unlikely that you will contract the disease again.

You might not have been immunized against some of the childhood diseases. If you are not sure about which immunizations you have received or need, contact your doctor.

## ◆ PROTECTING YOURSELF FROM DISEASE TRANSMISSION

### The Exposure Control Plan

Preventing infectious disease begins with preparation and planning. An Exposure Control Plan is an important step in removing or reducing employee exposure to blood and other possibly infectious materials. The Exposure Control Plan is the way in which an employer creates a system to protect its employees from infection. It is a key provision of the OSHA standard. The plan requires the employer to identify who will receive training, protective equipment, and vaccination.

An Exposure Control Plan should contain the following elements:

- Exposure determination
- The schedule and method of implementing other parts of the OSHA standard (that is, ways of meeting the requirements and recordkeeping)
- The procedures for evaluating details of an exposure incident

Exposure determination is one of the key elements of the Exposure Control Plan. It includes identifying and making a written record of jobs where exposure to blood can occur. The determination should be made without regard to using personal protective equipment.

The Exposure Control Plan should be placed where employees can easily use it and must be updated each year or more often if changes in exposure occur.

Because of an increase in complaints about occupational exposure to TB, OSHA has begun to enforce policies and procedures for occupational exposure to tuberculosis in workplace settings where workers have a greater incidence of TB infection. These include—

* health care settings
* correctional institutions
* homeless shelters
* long-term care facilities for the elderly
* drug treatment centers

Employers are required to provide employees with information and training regarding hazards of TB transmission, signs and symptoms, medical surveillance, and therapy and site-specific protocols, including the purpose and proper use of engineering and work practice controls. Although not part of the bloodborne pathogen standard, you should be aware of TB-related regulations that may affect your workplace.

## Immunizations

Preventing infectious diseases begins with maintaining good health and always practicing good personal hygiene, such as washing hands frequently (Fig. 3-7). You should also be immunized against several diseases. The following immunizations are recommended:

* DPT (diphtheria, pertussis, tetanus)
* Polio
* Hepatitis B
* MMR (measles, mumps, rubella)
* Influenza

Check with your doctor to see whether you need any boosters to keep your immunizations up to date.

The OSHA standard requires an employer to make the hepatitis B vaccination series available to all employees who have job expo-

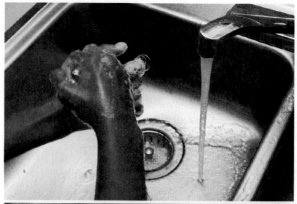
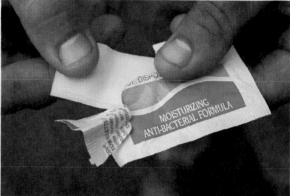
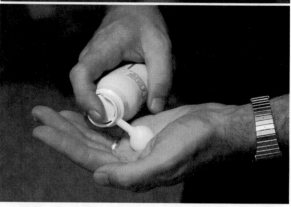

**Figure 3-7** Thorough handwashing after giving care helps protect you against disease.

sure to blood or other body fluids. It also requires post-exposure evaluation and follow-up to employees who have an exposure incident.

The employer shall make sure that all medical evaluations and procedures, including the hepatitis B vaccination series and post-exposure evaluation and follow-up, are—

* Made available at no cost to the employee.
* Made available to employees at a reasonable time and place.
* Provided by or under the supervision of a li-

censed physician or health care professional. People getting vaccinations should be carefully watched for at least 30 minutes after injection. Approximately 10 percent of all individuals will have an allergic reaction to the vaccine.

♦ Provided according to the current recommendations of the U.S. Public Health Office.

OSHA has also added special considerations for employees who provide first aid for incidents occuring in the workplace. OSHA believes there is a low risk of exposure for these first aiders. The option of post-exposure prevention measures, including hepatitis B vaccination within 24 hours of exposure, is now available. OSHA believes that this option will minimize the risk to employees and lessen demands on limited supplies of the vaccine.

This option applies to employees whose routine work assignment does not include administering first aid. It does not apply to employees who provide first aid at a first aid station, clinic, or dispensary or to health care, emergency response, or public safety personnel expected to provide first aid in the course of their work.

OSHA considers the selection of this option a technical violation of the standard, but does not impose any penalty on the employer. However, the following conditions must be met:

♦ The exposure control plan must include reporting procedures for first aid incidents involving exposure. The procedures must ensure that incidents are reported before the end of the shift in which they occur.

♦ Reports of first aid incidents must include the names of all first aiders involved and the details of the incident. The report must also include the date and time of the incident and if an exposure incident has occurred.

♦ Exposure reports must be included on lists of first aid incidents. They must be readily available to employees and provided to OSHA on request.

♦ First aid providers must be trained under the bloodborne pathogens standard that covers the reporting procedure specifics.

♦ All first aiders who provide assistance in any incident involving blood or other potentially infectious materials, regardless of whether a specific exposure incident occurs, must be offered the full hepatitis B vaccination series. This immunization should be offered as soon as possible, but in no event later than 24 hours following exposure. If an exposure incident occurs, other post-exposure follow-up procedures must be initiated immediately.

## Precautions

Sometimes we might like to vary the level of protection we use based on what a person looks like, the circumstances surrounding the incident, or where he or she is at the time of the incident. However, the world is not that simple. Very often you will not know the health status of the people you work with or care for. The one time you stop being careful may be the very time that you become infected by someone who does not fit your notion of people who are likely to be infected.

The Center for Disease Control and Prevention has identified precautions taken to prevent occupational-risk exposure to blood and other body fluids containing visible blood as **universal precautions.** Precautions taken to isolate or prevent the risk of exposure from any other type of bodily substance are known as **body substance isolation (BSI).** Regardless of the type of exposure risk, you must follow basic precautions and safe practices each time you prepare to provide care. These precautions and practices include the following four areas—

♦ Personal hygiene
♦ Personal protective equipment
♦ Engineering and work practice controls
♦ Equipment cleaning and disinfecting.

Maintaining good personal hygiene habits, such as frequent hand washing and proper grooming, are two important ways to prevent

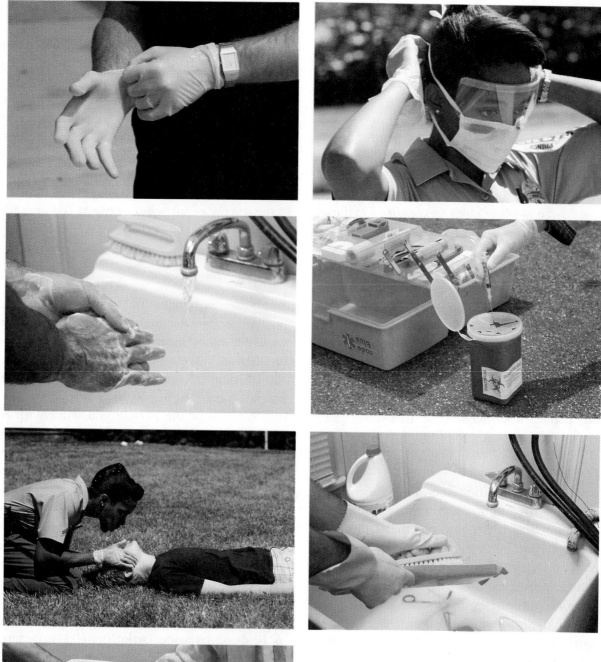

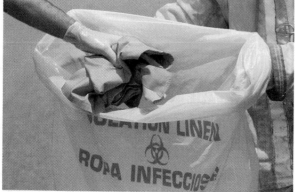

**Figure 3-8** Following basic precautions decreases your risk of contracting or transmitting an infection.

disease transmission regardless of any personal protective equipment you might use. Infection control products, such as waterless antiseptic hand cleansers now available, even allow you to clean your hands when soap and water are not readily available. These simple methods of infection control can help prevent bacteria or germs that may come in contact with the skin from contracting or transmitting an infectious disease (Fig. 3-8). By following good personal hygiene practices you greatly reduce your chances of disease transmission.

## Protective Equipment

Personal protective equipment (PPE) includes all equipment and supplies that keep you from direct contact with infected materials. These include disposable gloves, gowns, masks and shields, protective eyeware, and resuscitation devices (Table 3-3). To minimize your risk of contracting or transmitting an infectious disease, follow these guidelines for the use of protective equipment.

* Wear disposable (single-use) gloves, when it is possible you will contact blood or body fluids. This may happen directly through contact with a victim or indirectly through contact with soiled clothing or other personal articles.
* Remove gloves by turning them inside out, beginning at the wrist and peeling them off. When removing the second glove, do not touch the soiled surfaces with your bare hand. Hook the inside of the glove at the wrist and peel the glove off.
* Discard discolored, torn, or punctured gloves.
* Do not clean or reuse disposable (single-use) gloves.
* Avoid handling items such as pens, combs, or radios when wearing soiled gloves.
* Change gloves when you give care to different persons.
* In addition to gloves, wear protective coverings, such as a mask, eyewear, and gown, whenever you are likely to contact blood or other body fluids that may splash.
* Cover any cuts, scrapes, or skin irritations prior to putting on protective clothing.
* Use breathing devices such as disposable resuscitation masks and airway devices.
* Use a NIOSH-approved high efficiency particulate-air (HEPA) respirator if you are likely to be exposed to TB or other airborne pathogens.

## Personal Hygiene

Your personal hygiene habits are as important in preventing infection as any equipment you might use. These habits and practices can prevent any materials that might have gotten through the protective equipment from staying in contact with your body. Following certain guidelines for personal hygiene can greatly cut down your risk of contracting or transmitting an infectious disease:

* Wash your hands thoroughly with soap and water immediately after providing care. Use a utility or restroom sink, not one in a food preparation area.
* Avoid eating, drinking, and touching your mouth, nose, or eyes while providing care or before washing hands.

## Engineering and Work Practice Controls

Engineering controls are controls that isolate or remove the hazard from the workplace. Engineering controls include puncture-resistant containers for sharp equipment and mechanical needle recapping devices. Once put in place, engineering controls should be examined and maintained or replaced periodically.

Work practice controls reduce the likelihood of exposure by changing the way a task is carried out. The protection provided by work practice controls is based on the way an employer and employee behave rather than on a physical device.

Engineering and work practice controls are

**Table 3-3** Recommended Protective Equipment Against HIV and HBV Transmission in Prehospital Settings

| Task or activity | Disposable gloves | Gown | Mask | Protective eyewear |
|---|---|---|---|---|
| Bleeding control with spurting blood | Yes | Yes | Yes | Yes |
| Bleeding control with minimal bleeding | Yes | No | No | No |
| Emergency childbirth | Yes | Yes | Yes, if splash likely | Yes, if splash likely |
| Helping with intravenous (IV) line | Yes | No | No | No |
| Oral/nasal suctioning manually clearing airway | Yes | No | No, unless splash likely | No, unless splash likely |
| Handling and cleaning contaminated equipment and clothing | Yes | No, unless soiling likely | No | No |

Excerpt from Department of Health and Human Services, Public Health Services: *A curriculum guide for public safety and emergency response workers prevention of transmission immunodeficiency virus and hepatitis B virus,* Atlanta, Georgia, February 1989, Dept. Health and Human Services, Centers for Disease Control.

established to ensure good industrial hygiene. Adhering to these controls minimizes the risk of exposure in the work place.

◆ Avoid needlestick injuries by not trying to bend or recap any needles.

◆ Place sharp items (for example, needles, scalpel blades) in puncture-resistant, leak-proof, labeled containers.

◆ Perform all procedures in a way that cuts down on splashing, spraying, splattering, and producing droplets of blood or other potentially infectious materials.

◆ Remove bloodied, soiled protective clothing as soon as possible.

◆ Clean and disinfect all equipment and work surfaces possibly soiled by blood or other body fluids.

◆ Wash your hands thoroughly with soap and water immediately after providing care. Use a utility or restroom sink, not one in a food preparation area.

◆ Avoid eating, drinking, smoking, applying cosmetics or lip balm, handling contact lenses, and touching the mouth, nose, or eyes in work areas where an exposure to infectious materials may occur.

◆ Make hand washing facilities readily accessible to employees' work areas.

◆ Provide antiseptic towelettes or hand cleanser where hand washing facilities are not available.

◆ Ensure all sharp instrument disposal containers are—
  ◆ puncture resistant
  ◆ labeled or color-coded
  ◆ leak proof
  ◆ able to prevent access to contents

## Equipment Cleaning and Disinfecting

It is important to clean and disinfect equipment to prevent infections. Handle all soiled equipment, supplies, or other materials with great care until they are properly cleaned and disinfected. Place all disposable items that are contaminated in labeled containers. Place all soiled clothing in properly marked plastic bags for disposal or washing.

To disinfect equipment soiled with blood or body fluids, wash thoroughly with a solution of common household chlorine bleach and water. Approximately ¼ cup of bleach per gallon of water is enough. Surfaces, such as floors, woodwork, ambulance and automobile seats, and countertops, must be cleaned of any visible soil before using a bleach solution.

Wash and dry protective clothing and work uniforms according to the manufacturer's instructions. Scrub soiled boots, leather shoes, and other leather goods, such as belts, with soap, a brush, and hot water.

Biohazard warning labels are required on any container or equipment that has been or is potentially contaminated with infectious materials (Fig. 3-9). Signs should be posted at entrances of work areas where potentially infectious material may be present. Biohazard signs and labels should be fluorescent orange, orange-red, or predominantly so with lettering or symbols in a contrasting color such as black. Red bags or red containers may be substituted for labels.

If an incident occurs, that creates disposable waste or soiled laundry, the employer should provide containers to store the materials until they are disposed of or laundered. The containers must have warning labels or signs, such as "biohazard," to eliminate or minimize exposure of employees. In addition, the employer must provide training to ensure that all employees understand and avoid the hazard.

The OSHA standard requires that the employer keep the work area clean and sanitary. The employer is required to develop and put into action a written schedule for cleaning and decontamination at the work site. The schedule should be based on the location in the facility, the type of surface to be cleaned, the

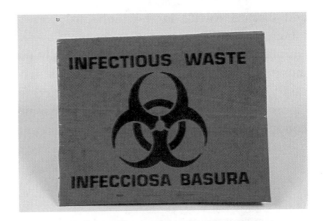

**Figure 3-9** Biohazard warning label.

type of soil present, and the task or procedures being done.

In addition, the employer has a responsibility to have a plan in place to deal with any spill that might occur. The plan should include a system to report the spill, and the action taken to resolve the spill. It should also include a list of employees responsible for containment, instructions for cleanup, and the final disposition of the spill.

The first step in dealing with a spill is containment. Spill containment units designed for hazardous materials are sold and work very well. However, any absorbent material, such as paper towels, can be used if the material is disposed of properly.

The steps for spill management are as follows:

- Wear gloves and other appropriate personal protective equipment when cleaning spills.
- Clean up spills immediately, or as soon as possible after the spill occurs.
- If the spill is mixed with sharp objects, such as broken glass and needles, do not pick these up with your hands. Use tongs, broom and dustpan, or two pieces of cardboard.
- Dispose of the absorbent material used to collect the spill in a labeled biohazard container.
- Flood the area with disinfectant solution, and allow it to stand for at least 20 minutes.
- Use paper towels to absorb the solution,

and discard towels in the biohazard container.

Following these precautions will usually remove at least one of the four conditions necessary for disease transmission as depicted in Figure 3-3 on p. 32. Remember, if only one condition is missing, infection will not occur.

## ♦ IF AN EXPOSURE OCCURS

If you suspect you have been exposed to an infectious disease, wash any area of contact as quickly as possible, and write down what happened. Exposures usually involve contact with potentially infectious blood or other fluids through a needle stick, broken or scraped skin, or the mucous membranes of the eyes, nose, or mouth. Inhaling potentially infected airborne droplets also may be an exposure. Most employers have **protocols** (standardized methods) for reporting infectious disease exposure.

Protocols should include the following elements:
- List of events included in the protocol
- List of immediate actions to be taken by exposed employee to reduce the chances of infection
- When or how quickly the employee should report the exposure incident
- Where and to whom the employee should report the exposure incident
- Which forms the employee should complete
- Directions for investigating the incident
- Medical follow-up that would include post-exposure vaccination

If you think you have been exposed to an infectious disease, it is your responsibility to notify your supervisor immediately. A test may be done to see if the material was in fact infected. But even before a disease is confirmed, you should receive medical evaluation, counseling, and post-exposure care, such as the hepatitis B vaccine. Your supervisor or medical personnel is responsible for notifying any other personnel who might have been exposed. If your system does not have a designated physician or nurse at a local hospital for follow-up care, see your personal physician.

## ♦ SUMMARY

Although the body's natural defense system defends well against disease, pathogens can still enter the body and sometimes cause infection. These pathogens can be transmitted in four ways: by direct contact with an infected person; by indirect contact with a soiled object; by inhaling air exhaled by an infected person; and through a bite from an infected animal, insect, or even a person.

Infectious diseases that you should be aware of include hepatitis, herpes, meningitis, tuberculosis, and HIV infection, including AIDS. You should know how the diseases are transmitted and take appropriate measures to protect yourself from them. Remember that the four conditions of infection must be present for a disease to be transmitted.

The Occupational Safety and Health Administration (OSHA) has issued regulations for on-the-job exposure to bloodborne pathogens. The agency has determined that employees face a significant risk as a result of on-the-job exposure to blood and other potentially infectious materials because they may contain bloodborne pathogens. OSHA concludes that this hazard can be reduced or removed using a combination of engineering and work practice controls, personal protective clothing and equipment, training, medical surveillance, hepatitis B vaccination, signs and labels, and other provisions. The OSHA regulation defines the range of employees covered by the standard, and it sets forth certain requirements that employers must meet to maintain work sites in a clean and sanitary condition.

The regulations on bloodborne pathogens have placed specific responsibilities on employers for protection of employees. They include—

* Identifying positions or tasks covered by the standard.
* Creating an Exposure Control Plan to minimize the possibility of exposure.
* Using work practices, such as following precautions, to minimize the possibility of infection.
* Using engineering controls, such as puncture resistant containers for sharp objects, to minimize the possibility of infection.
* Creating a system for easy identification of soiled material and its disposal.
* Developing a system of annual training for all covered employees.
* Offering the opportunity for employees to

get counseling and medical care, such as the hepatitis B vaccination, at no cost.

* Establishing clear procedures to follow for reporting an exposure.
* Creating a system of record keeping that includes updates in protocols and Exposure Control Plans, employee training, employee medical records, and follow-up.

Following OSHA guidelines, especially the precautions, greatly decreases your risk of contracting or transmitting an infectious disease. If you suspect you have been exposed to such a disease, always document it or notify your supervisor and other involved personnel. Seek medical help and participate in any follow-up procedures.

## ♦ Review Questions ♦

**1.** The OSHA regulations apply to—
a. All employees at any workplace.
b. Employees who have on-the-job exposure to bacteria.
c. Employees who have on-the-job exposure to blood.
d. Employees in health care facilities only.

**2.** Direct contact transmission occurs when—
a. A person breathes in infected droplets.
b. A person is bitten by an infected animal or person.
c. A person contacts dressings and surfaces soiled with infected body fluids.
d. A person touches an infected person's body fluids.

**3.** Work-practice controls—
a. Change the way a task is carried out.
b. Include handwashing immediately after giving care.
c. Require that all equipment is cleaned and disinfected.
d. All of the above.

**4.** Which step should you take if you think you have been exposed to an infectious disease?
a. Notify your supervisor at once.
b. Go to a hospital emergency room.
c. Wash any area of contact as soon as possible.
d. a and c.

Answers. 1. c; 2. d; 3. d; 4. d

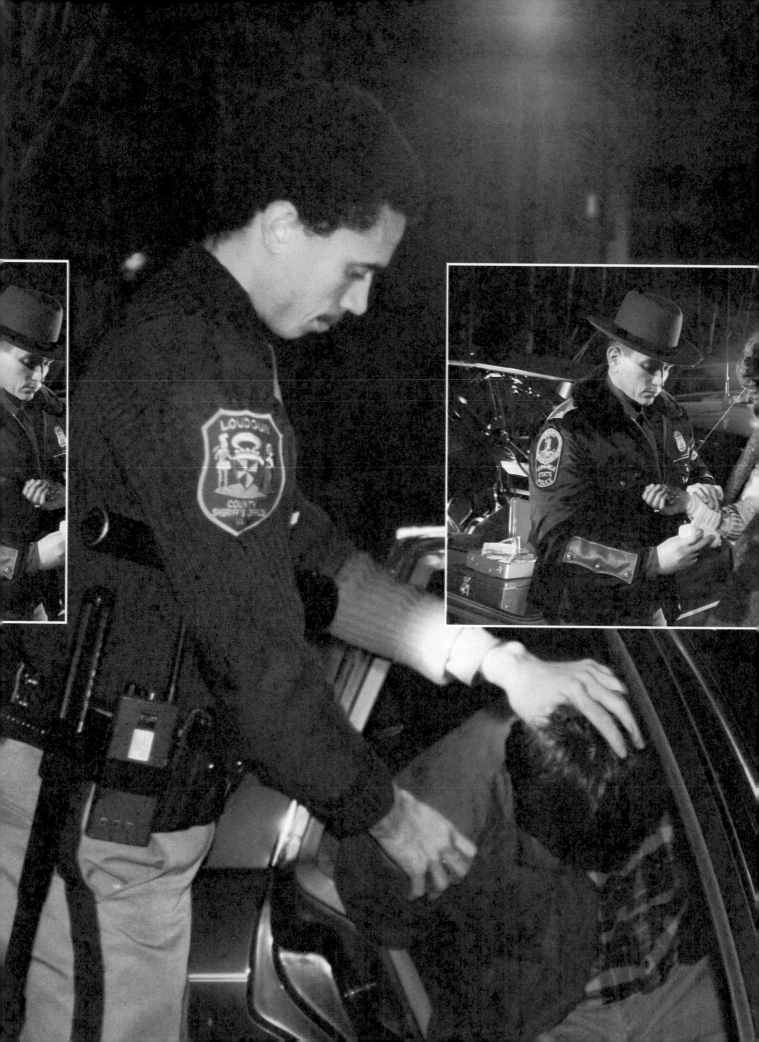

# Part Three

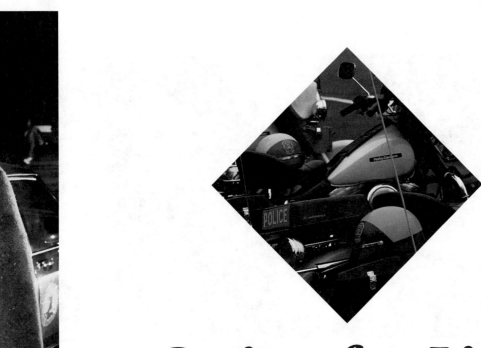

# Caring for Life-Threatening Emergencies

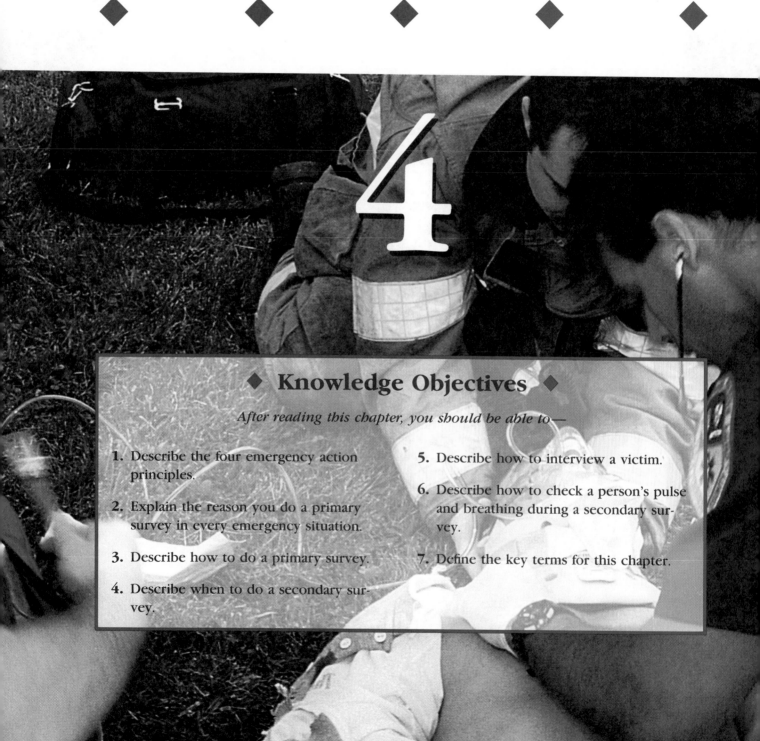

# Priorities of Care

**4**

## ◆ Knowledge Objectives ◆

*After reading this chapter, you should be able to—*

1. Describe the four emergency action principles.

2. Explain the reason you do a primary survey in every emergency situation.

3. Describe how to do a primary survey.

4. Describe when to do a secondary survey.

5. Describe how to interview a victim.

6. Describe how to check a person's pulse and breathing during a secondary survey.

7. Define the key terms for this chapter.

# ◆ Skill Objectives ◆

*After reading this chapter and completing the class activities, you should be able to—*

1. Demonstrate how to do a primary survey.

2. Make appropriate decisions about care when given an example of an emergency requiring you to do a primary survey.

# ◆ Key Terms ◆

**Brachial arteries:** Arteries located in each arm.

**Carotid arteries:** Arteries located in the neck that supply blood to the head and neck.

**Emergency action principles (EAPs):** Four steps to guide a rescuer's actions in any emergency.

**Primary survey:** A check for conditions that are an immediate threat to a victim's life.

**Secondary survey:** A check for injuries or conditions that could become life-threatening if not cared for.

**Signs:** Any observable evidence of injury or illness, such as bleeding or unusually pale skin.

**Symptoms:** Something the victim tells you about his or her condition, such as, "My head hurts," or "I am dizzy."

# ◆ Main Ideas ◆

1. The following four emergency action principles (EAPs) are your plan of action for any emergency situation:
   - Survey the scene.
   - Do a primary survey.
   - Summon additional medical personnel if necessary.
   - Do a secondary survey, if appropriate.

2. Always survey the scene to make sure it is safe and to try to determine what happened before you approach the victim.

3. Do not move the victim unless there is immediate danger.

4. In the primary survey, you check to see if the victim is conscious, has an open airway, is breathing, has a heartbeat, and is bleeding severely.

5. If the victim is conscious, interview the victim to find out if the victim has any signs or symptoms that indicate a potential life-threatening condition such as a heart attack.

6. During the secondary survey, check the victim's breathing and pulse rate.

## ◆ INTRODUCTION

In this chapter you will learn a plan of action to guide you through any emergency. When an emergency occurs, you may at first feel confused. But you can train yourself to remain calm and think before you act. Ask yourself, "What do I need to do? How can I help most effectively?" The four **emergency action principles (EAPs)** answer these questions and are the plan of action for any emergency.

## ◆ EMERGENCY ACTION PRINCIPLES

The EAPs are—

1. Survey the scene.
2. Do a **primary survey** to identify and care for immediate life-threatening conditions.
3. Summon additional medical personnel if necessary.
4. Do a **secondary survey** to identify and care for any additional problems, if appropriate.

These principles, conducted in this order, can ensure your safety and that of the victim and bystanders. They will also increase the victim's chance of survival if he or she has a serious illness or injury.

## Step One: Survey the Scene

Once you recognize that an emergency has occurred and decide to act, you must make sure the scene of the emergency is safe for you, the victim(s), and any bystanders. Take time to survey the scene and answer these questions:

1. Is the scene safe?
2. What happened?
3. How many victims are there?
4. Can bystanders help?

### Before You Approach the Victim

When you survey the scene, look for anything that may threaten your safety and that of the victim and bystanders. Dangers include downed power lines, traffic, fire, unstable structures, and deep or swift-moving water. Take the necessary precautions when working in a dangerous environment. If you are not properly trained and do not have the necessary equipment, do not approach the victim. Summon the necessary personnel.

Nothing is gained by risking your own safety. An emergency that begins with one victim could end up with two if you are hurt. If you suspect the scene is unsafe, wait and watch until the necessary personnel and equipment arrive. If conditions change, you may then be able to approach the victim.

### As You Approach the Victim

Try to find out what happened. Look around the scene for clues to what caused the emergency and the extent of the damage. Doing this will cause you to think about the possible type and extent of the victim's injuries. You may discover a situation that requires you to act immediately. As you approach the victim, take in the whole picture. Nearby objects, such as shattered glass, a fallen ladder, or a spilled medicine container, may suggest what happened (Fig. 4-1). If the victim is unconscious, surveying the scene may be the only way you can determine what happened.

When you survey the scene, look carefully for more than one victim. You may not see everyone at first. For example, in a vehicle collision, an open door may be a clue that a victim has left the car or was thrown from it. If one victim is bleeding or screaming loudly, you may overlook another victim who is unconscious. It is also easy in any emergency situation to overlook an infant or small child. Always look for more than one victim. Ask anyone present how many people may be involved. If you find more than one victim, ask bystanders to help you provide care.

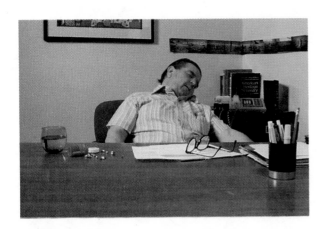

**Figure 4-1** If the victim is unconscious, nearby objects may be your only clue to what has happened.

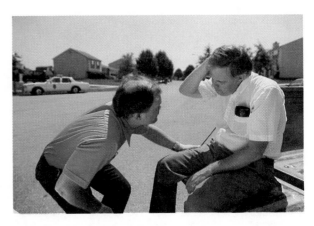

**Figure 4-2** When talking to the victim, position yourself close to the victim's eye level and speak in a calm and positive manner.

Look for bystanders who can help. Bystanders may be able to tell you what happened or help in other ways. A bystander who knows the victim may know whether he or she has any medical conditions or allergies. Bystanders can meet and direct additional personnel to your location, help keep the area free of unnecessary traffic, and help you provide care.

### Once You Reach the Victim

Once you reach the victim, quickly survey the scene again to see if it is still safe. At this point, you may see other dangers, clues to what happened, and victims or bystanders that you did not notice before.

*You respond to an automobile crash. A car has veered off the road and landed in a ditch. After surveying the scene and deciding it is safe to approach, you move to the car. As you come closer, you see a woman lying motionless on the ground near the car. But you also smell gasoline. What should you do? Is there a danger? Should you move her away from the car or try to care for her there?*

As a rule, do not move a victim unless there is an immediate danger such as a fire, poisonous fumes, or an unstable structure. The odor of gasoline by itself is not sufficient cause to move the victim. If the area is dangerous and

the victim does not seem to be seriously injured, ask the victim to move to safety where you can help him or her. If the area is dangerous and the victim cannot move, you may try to move the victim as quickly as possible without making his or her condition worse. If there is no immediate danger, tell the victim not to move.

When you reach the victim, try not to alarm him or her. Try to position yourself close to the victim's eye level (Fig. 4-2). Speak in a calm and positive manner. Identify yourself to a conscious victim and advise him or her that you are there to help.

### Step Two: Do a Primary Survey

In every emergency situation, you first must determine if conditions exist that are an immediate threat to the victim's life. You will discover these conditions by looking for **signs,** observable evidence of injury or illness. You discover the signs of life-threatening conditions in the primary survey. You check to see if the victim—

- ♦ Is conscious.
- ♦ Has an open airway.
- ♦ Is breathing.
- ♦ Has a heartbeat.
- ♦ Is bleeding severely.

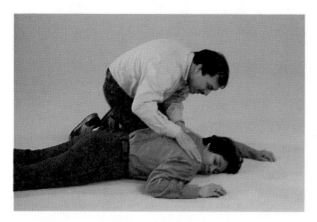

**Figure 4-3** Determine if the person is conscious by gently tapping and asking, "Are you okay?"

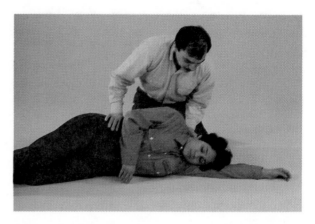

**Figure 4-4** If the victim's position prevents you from checking the ABCs, roll the victim gently onto his or her back.

The primary survey takes only seconds to perform.

Begin the primary survey by determining if the victim is conscious. Do this by gently tapping him or her and asking, "Are you okay?" (Fig. 4-3). Do not jostle or move the victim. A victim who can speak or cry is conscious, breathing, and has a pulse.

If the victim is unable to respond, he or she may be unconscious. Unconsciousness can indicate a life-threatening condition. When a person is unconscious, the tongue relaxes and may fall to the back of the throat, blocking the airway. This can cause breathing to stop. Soon after, the heart will stop beating. Therefore, the next thing you must do is to check the victim's airway, breathing, and circulation.

Remembering these steps is easy. The three steps are called the ABCs of the primary survey.

> **A** = *Airway*
> **B** = *Breathing*
> **C** = *Circulation*

If you can, try to check the ABCs in whatever position you find the victim, especially if you suspect the victim has a head or spine injury. Sometimes, however, the victim's position prevents you from checking the ABCs. In this case, you should roll the victim gently onto his or her back, keeping the head and spine in as straight a line as possible (Fig. 4-4).

## Check the Airway

Be sure the victim has an open airway, the pathway for air from the mouth and nose to the lungs. Without an open airway, the victim cannot breathe. Remember, a victim who can speak or cry is conscious, has an open airway, is breathing, and has a pulse.

Determining if an unconscious victim has an open airway is more difficult. To open an unconscious victim's airway, tilt the head back and lift the chin (Fig. 4-5). This action moves the tongue away from the back of the throat, allowing air to enter the lungs. For someone you suspect has a head or spine injury, you modify the technique, as you will learn in Chapter 5. After opening the airway, check for breathing.

Sometimes, opening the airway does not result in a free passage of air. This happens when a victim's airway is blocked by liquid, food, or other objects. In this case, you will need to remove the obstruction. Chapter 5 describes how to care for an obstructed airway.

## Check Breathing

If the victim is breathing, the chest will rise and fall. But if the victim is unconscious, you

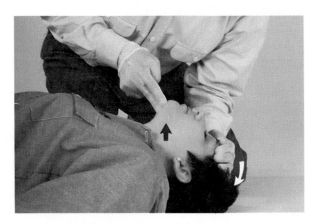

**Figure 4-5** Tilt the head and lift the chin to open the airway.

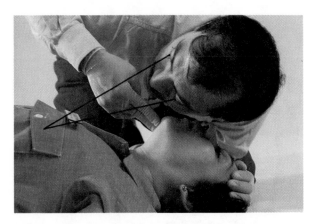

**Figure 4-6** To check breathing, look, listen, and feel for breathing for about 5 seconds.

must look, listen, and feel for signs of breathing. Position yourself so you can hear and feel air as it escapes from the victim's nose and mouth. At the same time, watch the rise and fall of the chest. Take the time to look, listen, and feel for breathing for about 5 seconds (Fig. 4-6).

If the victim is not breathing, you must breathe for him or her. Begin by giving 2 slow breaths. This will get air into the victim's lungs. The longer a victim goes without oxygen, the more likely he or she is to die. This process of breathing for the victim is called **rescue breathing.** You will learn how to give rescue breathing in Chapter 5.

### Check Circulation

The last step in the primary survey is checking for the circulation of blood. If the heart has stopped, blood will not circulate throughout the body. If blood does not circulate, the victim will die in just a few minutes because the brain will not receive any oxygen.

If a person is breathing, his or her heart is beating and is circulating blood. If the victim is not breathing, you must find out whether his or her heart is beating by checking the pulse. In the primary survey, you feel for an adult's or child's pulse at either of the **carotid arteries** located in the neck (Fig. 4-7).

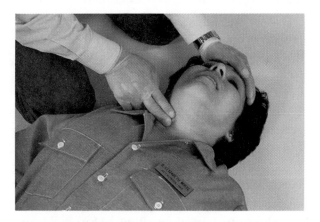

**Figure 4-7** Determine if the heart is beating by feeling for a carotid pulse at either side of the neck.

To find the pulse, feel for the Adam's apple at the front of the neck, then slide your fingers into the groove at the side of the neck. Sometimes the pulse may be difficult to find, since it may be slow or weak. If at first you do not find a pulse, relocate the Adam's apple and **again** slide your fingers into place. When you think you are in the right spot, take 5 to 10 seconds to feel for the pulse. To find an **infant's** pulse, you place your fingers over the **brachial artery,** located on the inside of the upper arm, midway between the shoulder and elbow (Fig. 4-8).

If the victim does not have a pulse, you need to keep oxygen-rich blood circulating.

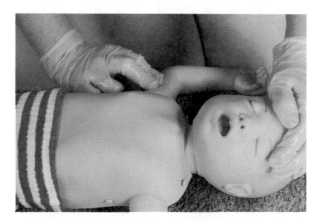

**Figure 4-8** To find an infant's pulse, feel for the brachial artery in the upper arm.

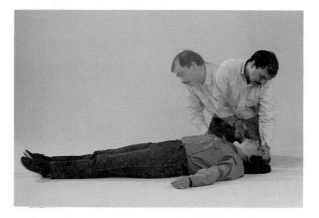

**Figure 4-9** Visually check for signs of severe bleeding by looking from head to toe.

This involves doing rescue breathing to get oxygen into the victim's lungs and chest compressions to circulate the oxygen to the brain. This procedure is called cardiopulmonary resuscitation (CPR) and is described in Chapter 7.

Checking circulation also means looking for severe bleeding. Bleeding is severe when blood spurts from the wound or cannot be controlled. It is life-threatening. Check for severe bleeding by looking from head to toe for signs of external bleeding (Fig. 4-9). Severe bleeding must be controlled before you provide any further care.

If you must leave the victim for any reason, such as to call your emergency number, place him or her in the recovery position to help keep the airway open (Fig. 4-10). Place the victim on one side, bend the top leg and move it forward to hold the victim in that position. Support the head so that the face is angled toward the ground. In this position, if the victim vomits, the airway will stay clear.

## Step Three: Summon Additional Personnel

You may feel the victim needs the benefit of additional medical personnel or equipment. As a general rule, first responders such as fire fighters or law enforcement personnel should summon more advanced medical personnel to

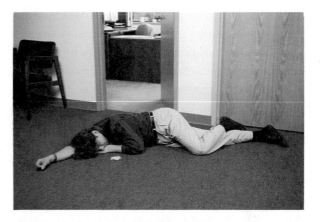

**Figure 4-10** Place an unconscious victim in the recovery position if you must leave for any reason.

the scene if any of the following conditions exists:

- Unconsciousness or altered level of consciousness (semiconsciousness, disorientation)
- Breathing problems (difficulty breathing or no breathing)
- Persistent chest or abdominal pain or pressure
- No pulse
- Severe bleeding
- Vomiting blood or passing blood
- Suspected poisoning
- Seizures, severe headache, slurred speech
- Suspected or obvious injuries to head or spine

◆ Suspected broken bones
◆ Severe burns

## Step Four: Do a Secondary Survey

Once you are certain that the victim has no life-threatening conditions, you can begin the fourth EAP, the secondary survey. The secondary survey is a systematic method of gathering additional information about injuries or conditions that may need care. These conditions or injuries may not be immediately life-threatening but could become so if not cared for. If, however, you find life-threatening conditions, such as unconsciousness, no breathing, no pulse, or severe bleeding, during the primary survey, do not waste time with a secondary survey. Instead, provide care only for the life-threatening conditions.

The secondary survey has three basic steps:

1. Interview the victim and bystanders.
2. Check vital signs (such as the rate and quality of pulse and breathing, skin color and temperature, blood pressure, and pupil reaction).
3. Do a head-to-toe examination.

If the victim is able to speak, interview the victim to try to learn if he or she has any signs or symptoms, such as difficulty breathing or chest pain, that indicate a condition that could become life-threatening at any moment, such as a heart attack. Also check the victim's pulse and breathing.

When possible, write down the information you find during the secondary survey. Sometimes you may need to have someone else write down the information or help you remember it. You can give this information to other medical personnel when requested. Your information may help determine what type of medical care the victim will receive later.

As you do the secondary survey, try not to move the victim. Most injured people will find the most comfortable position for themselves. For example, a person with chest pain who is having trouble breathing may be sitting upright. Let the victim continue to sit upright. Do not ask him or her to change positions.

### Interview the Victim and Bystanders

Begin by asking the victim and bystanders simple questions to learn more about what happened and the victim's condition. This procedure should not take much time. You are not only looking for signs of the victim's condition but also for symptoms. A **symptom** is something the victim tells you about his or her condition, such as, "I am dizzy," or "My chest hurts."

If you have not done so already, remember to identify yourself and to get the victim's consent before helping. Begin the interview by asking the victim's name. Using his or her name will make the victim more comfortable. Ask the following questions:

1. What happened?
2. Do you feel any pain anywhere?
3. Do you have any medical conditions?
4. Are you taking any **medication?**
5. Do you have any allergies?

If the victim has pain, ask him or her to describe it. You can expect to get descriptions such as burning, crushing, aching, or sharp pain. Ask when the pain started. Ask how bad the pain is.

Sometimes the victim will be unable to give you the information. This is often the case with a child or with an adult who has momentarily lost consciousness, or who is disoriented, and may not be able to recall what has happened. These victims may be frightened. Be calm and patient. Speak normally and in simple terms. Offer reassurance. Ask family members, friends, or bystanders what happened (Fig. 4-11). They may be able to give you helpful information, such as telling you if a victim has a medical condition you should

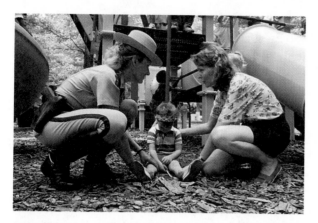

**Figure 4-11** Parents or other adults may be able to provide information about a child who is sick or injured.

be aware of. They may also be able to help calm the victim if necessary.

After you interview the victim, assess the victim's vital signs. Pulse and breathing are particularly important.

## Checking Vital Signs

With every heartbeat a wave of blood moves through the blood vessels. This creates a beat called the **pulse.** You can feel it with your fingertips in arteries near the skin. In the primary survey you are only concerned with whether a pulse is present. To determine this, you check the carotid arteries. In the secondary survey you are to determine pulse rate and quality, which is most often done by checking the **radial pulse** located on the thumb side of the wrist.

When the heart is healthy, it beats with a steady rhythm. This beat creates a regular pulse. A normal pulse for an adult is between 60 and 100 beats per minute. A well-conditioned athlete may have a pulse of 50 beats per minute or lower. If the heartbeat changes, so does the pulse. An abnormal pulse may be a sign of a potential problem. These signs include—

♦ Irregular pulse.
♦ Weak and hard-to-find pulse.
♦ Excessively fast or slow pulse.

When severely injured or unhealthy, the heart may beat unevenly, producing an irregular pulse. The rate at which the heart beats can also change. The pulse speeds up when a person is excited, anxious, in pain, losing blood, or under stress. It slows down when a person is relaxed. Some heart conditions can also speed up or slow down the pulse rate. Sometimes changes may be very subtle and difficult to detect. The most important change to note is a pulse that changes from being present to no pulse at all.

To check a pulse, place 2 fingers on top of a major artery where it is located close to the skin's surface. Pulse sites that are easy to locate are the carotid arteries in the neck, the radial artery in the wrist, and, for infants, the brachial artery in the upper arm (Fig. 4-12, *A-C*). To check the pulse rate, count the number of heartbeats that occur in 15 seconds and multiply that number by 4. The resulting number is the number of heartbeats per minute.

A sick or injured person's pulse may be hard to find. If you have trouble finding a pulse, keep checking for one periodically. Take your time. Remember, if a person is breathing, his or her heart is also beating. However, there may be a loss in circulation to one area, causing a loss of pulse. If you cannot find the pulse in one place, check it in another major artery (Fig. 4-13).

A healthy person breathes regularly, quietly, and effortlessly. The normal breathing rate for an adult is between 12 and 20 breaths per minute. However, some people breathe slightly slower or faster. Excitement, fear, or exercise will cause breathing to increase and become deeper. Certain injuries or illnesses can also cause both the breathing rate and quality to change.

During the secondary survey watch and listen for any changes in breathing. Abnormal breathing may indicate a potential problem. The signs and symptoms of abnormal breathing include—

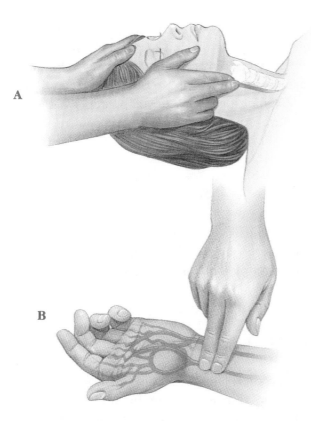

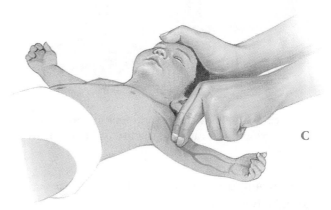

**Figure 4-12** A pulse can be checked in arteries that circulate close to the surface, such as **A,** the carotid artery, **B,** the radial artery, and, **C,** for infants, the brachial artery.

◆ Gasping for air.
◆ Noisy breathing, including whistling sounds, high-pitched noises, gurgling, or snoring.
◆ Excessively fast or slow breathing.
◆ Painful breathing.

Unlike the primary survey, in which you are concerned with whether a person is breathing at all, in the secondary survey you are concerned with the rate and quality of breathing. Look, listen, and feel again for breathing. Look for the rise and fall of the victim's chest or abdomen. Listen for the sounds as the person inhales and exhales. Count the number of times a person breathes (inhales or exhales) in 15 seconds; multiply that number by 4 to get the number of breaths per minute (Fig. 4-14). As you check for the rate and quality of breathing, try to do it without the victim's knowledge. If a victim realizes that you are checking his or her breathing, the victim may attempt to change his or her breathing pattern without being aware of doing so. Maintain the same position you were in when checking the pulse. In Chapter 5 you will learn more about

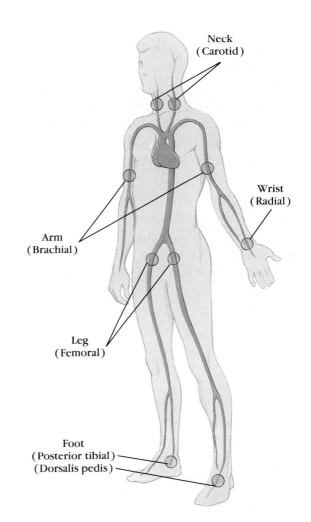

**Figure 4-13** Easily Located Pulse Sites

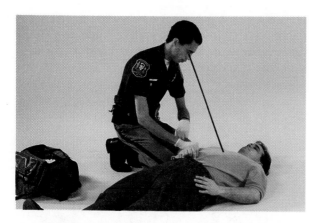

**Figure 4-14** Look, listen, and feel for breathing to determine the rate and quality of breathing.

the meaning of changes in breathing and the specific care to provide.

### Doing a Head-to-Toe Examination

The last step of the secondary survey is the head-to-toe examination. This step helps you gather additional information about the victim's condition. When you perform the head-to-toe examination, you generally begin checking the victim's head and finish at the toes. Use your senses—sight, sound, smell, and touch—to detect anything abnormal. For example, you may smell an unusual odor on the victim's breath that could indicate a diabetic problem. You may see pale skin or an unusual bruise or feel a deformed body part.

Pressing slightly on an area, such as the abdomen, could elicit a pain response from the victim. As you do this examination, watch for any changes in the victim's condition. If any life-threatening problems develop, stop whatever you are doing and provide care immediately for the problems.

### ◆ SUMMARY

When you respond to an emergency, follow the emergency action principles (EAPs). They provide a plan of action to guide you through any emergency. They also help to ensure your safety and the safety of any bystanders, as well. By following the EAPs, you will give a victim the best chance for survival.

- First, survey the scene for any possible dangers to yourself and any bystanders.
- Second, do a primary survey to check for any life-threatening problems with the victim's airway, breathing, and circulation.
- Third, summon additional medical personnel if necessary.
- Fourth, if you find no life-threatening conditions, do a secondary survey. Interview the victim to find out if the victim has any symptoms of conditions that could rapidly become life-threatening. Check pulse and breathing rate and provide appropriate care.

# ◆ Review Questions ◆

**1.** The emergency action principles provide—
a. Steps of care to follow in an emergency.
b. A plan to follow in any emergency.
c. Rules to follow to help advanced medical personnel when they arrive.
d. All of the above.

**2.** Why should you do a primary survey in every emergency situation?
a. Because it will protect you from legal liability
b. Because it identifies conditions that are an immediate threat to the victim's life
c. Because it enables you to protect the victim and bystanders from dangers at the scene
d. Because it is reassuring to the victim

**3.** If the victim is unconscious, the first thing you check is—
a. Circulation.
b. Heartbeat.
c. Airway.
d. Breathing.

**4.** After determining that a victim is unconscious and not breathing, which should you do next?
a. Check for a pulse.
b. Give two slow breaths.
c. Begin a secondary survey.
d. Control bleeding.

**5.** The purpose of the secondary survey is to—
a. Find injuries or conditions that are not immediately life-threatening.
b. Determine if the victim is bleeding severely.
c. Look for other victims you may not have noticed at first.
d. Find out if the victim has medical insurance.

**6.** When you interview the victim—
a. Spend a long time trying to determine what happened.
b. Be sure to have the victim lie down.
c. Ask the victim about any symptoms he or she may have.
d. All of the above.

**7.** When you check a victim's pulse in the secondary survey, you are trying to find out—
a. If the victim has a pulse.
b. If the victim is still breathing.
c. If the pulse is abnormal.
d. If the victim's arteries are damaged.

**Answers:** 1. b; 2. b; 3. c; 4. b; 5. a; 6. c; 7. c.

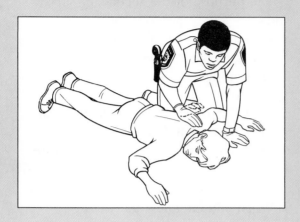

☐ **Check for consciousness**

♦ Tap or gently shake person.
♦ Shout, "Are you OK?"

**If person does not respond . . .**

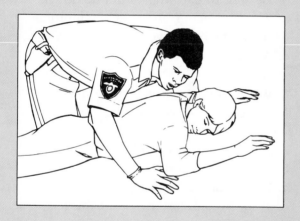

☐ **Check for breathing**

♦ Look, listen, and feel for about 5 seconds.

**If not breathing or you cannot tell . . .**

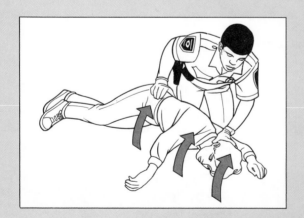

♦ Position victim onto back. Roll person as a single unit, while supporting the head and neck.

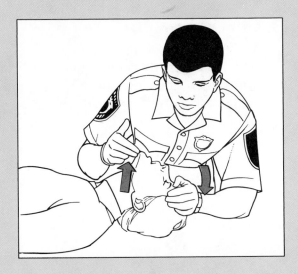

♦ Open the airway.
♦ Tilt head back and lift chin.

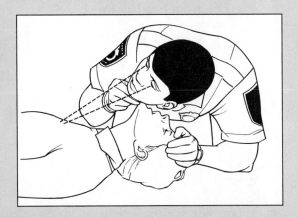

♦ Recheck breathing.
♦ Look, listen, and feel for about 5 seconds.

**If person is not breathing . . .**

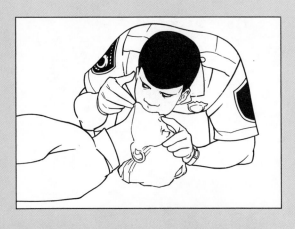

♦ Keep head tilted back.
♦ Pinch nose shut.
♦ Seal your lips tightly around person's mouth.
♦ Give 2 slow breaths, each lasting about 1½ seconds.
♦ Watch chest to see that the breaths go in.

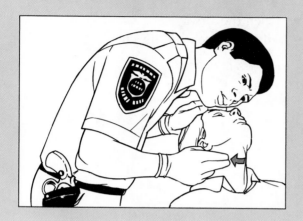

☐ **Check for a pulse**

 ◆ Locate Adam's apple.
 ◆ Slide fingers down into groove of neck on side closer to you.
 ◆ Feel for pulse for 5 to 10 seconds.

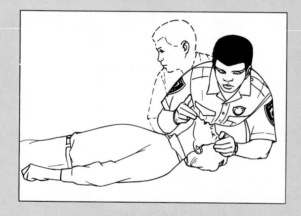

☐ **Check for severe bleeding**

 ◆ Look from head to toe for severe bleeding.

**If person has a pulse and is not breathing . . .**

 ◆ **Do rescue breathing.**

**If person does not have a pulse . . .**

 ◆ **Begin CPR.**

◆ **NOTES** ◆

# Breathing Emergencies

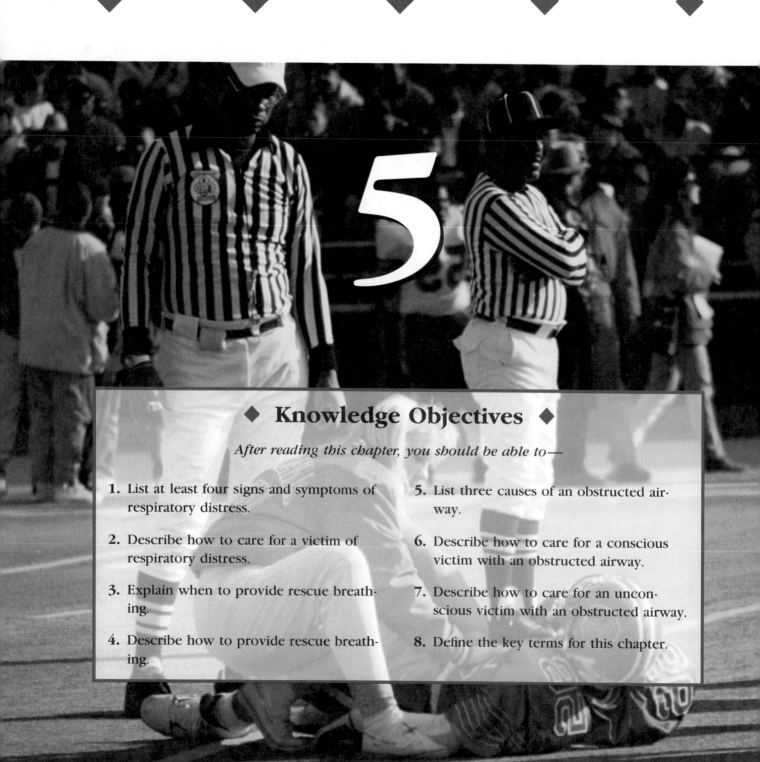

**5**

## ◆ Knowledge Objectives ◆

*After reading this chapter, you should be able to—*

1. List at least four signs and symptoms of respiratory distress.

2. Describe how to care for a victim of respiratory distress.

3. Explain when to provide rescue breathing.

4. Describe how to provide rescue breathing.

5. List three causes of an obstructed airway.

6. Describe how to care for a conscious victim with an obstructed airway.

7. Describe how to care for an unconscious victim with an obstructed airway.

8. Define the key terms for this chapter.

## ◆ Skill Objectives ◆

*After reading this chapter and completing the class activities, you should be able to—*

1. Demonstrate rescue breathing for an adult, a child, and an infant.
2. Demonstrate how to care for a conscious adult, child, and infant with an obstructed airway.
3. Demonstrate how to care for an unconscious adult, child, and infant with an obstructed airway.
4. Make appropriate decisions about care when given an example of an emergency in which a person is not breathing.

## ◆ Key Terms ◆

**Airway obstruction:** A blockage of the airway that prevents air from reaching a person's lungs.

**Aspiration:** Taking blood, vomit, saliva, or other foreign material into the lungs.

**Breathing emergency:** An emergency in which breathing is so impaired that life can be threatened.

**Finger sweep:** A technique used to remove foreign material from a victim's airway.

**Head-tilt/chin-lift:** A technique for opening the airway.

**Rescue breathing:** A technique of breathing for a nonbreathing victim.

**Respiratory arrest:** A condition in which breathing has stopped.

**Respiratory distress:** A condition in which breathing is difficult.

## ◆ Main Ideas ◆

1. Respiratory distress is the most common type of breathing emergency. The signs and symptoms of respiratory distress are usually obvious.
2. Providing care for respiratory distress is often the key to preventing respiratory arrest.
3. Rescue breathing is given to victims who are not breathing.
4. You will discover if you need to give rescue breathing during the primary survey.
5. For victims who are not breathing, give 1 breath every 5 seconds (adult), every 3 seconds (child), and every 3 seconds (infant).
6. Airway obstruction is a common cause of breathing emergencies.
7. Give abdominal thrusts if an adult or a child is choking. Give back blows and chest thrusts if an infant is choking.

## ♦ INTRODUCTION

In Chapter 2 you learned the parts of the airway and how the respiratory system functions. In Chapter 4 you learned that once you are sure the scene is safe, you begin a primary survey of the victim. The primary survey detects any life-threatening conditions. First check to see if the victim is conscious. Then complete the primary survey by checking the ABCs:

*A*irway
*B*reathing
*C*irculation

In this chapter you will learn how to care for breathing emergencies. Because oxygen is vital to life, you must always ensure that the victim has an open airway and is breathing. You will often detect a breathing emergency during the primary survey. In a **breathing emergency** a person's breathing is so impaired that life is threatened. This emergency can occur in two ways—breathing becomes difficult or breathing stops. A person who is having difficulty breathing is in **respiratory distress.** A person who has stopped breathing is in **respiratory arrest.**

Breathing emergencies can be caused by the following:

♦ An obstructed airway (choking)
♦ Illness, such as pneumonia
♦ Respiratory conditions, such as emphysema and asthma
♦ Electrocution
♦ Shock
♦ Near drowning
♦ Heart attack or heart disease
♦ Injury to the chest or lungs
♦ Allergic reactions, such as to food or to insect stings
♦ Drugs
♦ Poisoning, such as inhaling or ingesting toxic substances

## ♦ RESPIRATORY DISTRESS

Respiratory distress is the most common type of breathing emergency. It is not always caused by injuries or illness; it may result from excitement or anxiety.

### Signs and Symptoms of Respiratory Distress

The signs and symptoms of respiratory distress are usually obvious. Victims may look as if they cannot catch their breath, or they may gasp for air. Their breathing may be unusually fast, slow, deep, or shallow. They may make unusual noise, such as wheezing or gurgling or high-pitched, shrill sounds.

The victim's skin may also signal respiratory distress. At first, the skin may be unusually moist and appear flushed. Later, it may appear pale or bluish as the oxygen level in the blood falls. When the victim's skin or the nail beds of the fingers or toes appear blue, the condition is called *cyanosis.*

Victims may say they feel dizzy or lightheaded. They may feel pain in the chest and tingling in the hands and feet. They may be apprehensive or fearful. Any of these symptoms is a clue that the victim may be in respiratory distress. Table 5-1 lists the signs and symptoms of respiratory distress.

### Specific Types of Respiratory Distress

Although respiratory distress is often caused by injury, several other conditions also can cause it. These include asthma, emphysema, hyperventilation, and anaphylactic shock.

#### Asthma

**Asthma** is a condition that narrows the air passages and makes breathing difficult. During an asthma attack the air passages become constricted, or narrowed, by a spasm of the mus-

**Table 5-1** Signs and Symptoms of Respiratory Distress

| Conditions | Signs and symptoms |
|---|---|
| Abnormal breathing | Slow or rapid <br> Unusually deep or shallow <br> Victim is gasping for breath <br> Victim is wheezing, gurgling, or making high-pitched noises |
| Abnormal skin appearance | Unusually moist <br> Flushed, pale, ashen, or bluish appearance |
| How the victim feels | Short of breath <br> Dizzy or lightheaded <br> Chest pain or tingling in hands and feet |

cles lining the bronchi or by swelling of the bronchi themselves. Victims may become anxious or frightened because breathing is difficult.

Asthma is more common in children and young adults. It may be triggered by an allergic reaction to food, pollen, a drug, or an insect sting. Emotional stress may also trigger it. For some people, physical activity induces asthma. Normally, someone with asthma easily controls attacks with medication. These medications stop the muscle spasm, opening the airway and making breathing easier.

A characteristic sign of asthma is wheezing when exhaling, which occurs because air becomes trapped in the lungs. This trapped air may also make the victim's chest appear larger than normal, particularly in small children.

## Emphysema

**Emphysema** is a disease in which the lungs lose their ability to exchange carbon dioxide and oxygen effectively. Emphysema is often caused by smoking and usually develops over many years.

Victims suffer from shortness of breath. Exhaling is extremely difficult. They may cough and may have cyanosis or fever. Victims with advanced cases may be restless, confused, and weak and can go into respiratory or cardiac arrest. People with chronic (long-lasting or frequently recurring) emphysema will get worse over time.

## Hyperventilation

**Hyperventilation** occurs when someone breathes faster than normal. This rapid breathing upsets the body's balance of oxygen and carbon dioxide. Hyperventilation is often the result of fear or anxiety and is more likely to occur in people who are tense and nervous. However, it is also caused by injuries such as head injuries, by severe bleeding, or by conditions such as high fever, heart failure, lung disease, or diabetic emergencies. It can be triggered by asthma or exercise.

A characteristic sign of hyperventilation is shallow, rapid breathing. Despite their breathing efforts, victims say that they cannot get enough air or that they are suffocating. Therefore, they are often fearful and apprehensive or may appear confused. They may say they feel dizzy or that their fingers and toes feel numb or tingly.

## Anaphylactic Shock

*A woman is stung by a hornet at a company picnic. A colleague provided care for the sting and she returned to her activity. A few minutes later, she developed a rash and began to feel tightness in her chest and throat. When you arrive on the scene, she is having difficulty breathing. She states she feels her neck, face, and tongue beginning to swell. She is a victim of a life-threatening condition known as anaphylactic shock.*

**Anaphylactic shock,** also known as **anaphylaxis,** is a severe allergic reaction. The air passages may swell and restrict the victim's breathing. Anaphylaxis may be caused by insect stings, food, or medications such as penicillin. Some people know that they have a severe allergic reaction to certain substances. They may try to avoid these substances and may carry medication to reverse an allergic reaction.

The signs and symptoms of anaphylaxis can include a rash, a feeling of tightness in the chest and throat, and swelling of the face, neck, and tongue. The person may also feel dizzy or confused. Anaphylactic shock is a life-threatening emergency.

## Caring for Respiratory Distress

Recognizing the signs and symptoms of respiratory distress and providing emergency care are often the keys to preventing more serious emergencies. Respiratory distress may signal the beginning of a life-threatening condition. For example, it can be the first signal of a more serious breathing emergency or even a heart attack. Respiratory distress can lead to respiratory arrest, which, if not cared for, will result in death.

Many of the signs and symptoms of different types of respiratory distress are similar. You do not need to know the specific cause to provide care. If the victim is breathing, you know the heart is beating. Make sure the victim is not bleeding severely. Help him or her rest in a comfortable position. Usually, sitting is more comfortable than lying down because breathing is easier (Fig. 5-1). Reassure and comfort the victim. Have bystanders move back. Administer **supplemental oxygen** as soon as it is available.

When you are able, do a secondary survey. Remember that a victim experiencing breathing difficulty may have trouble talking. Talk to any bystanders who may know about the victim's problem. The victim can confirm answers of yes-or-no questions by nodding. If possible, reduce any anxiety; it may contribute to the victim's breathing difficulty. Help the victim take any prescribed medication, such as an **inhalant** (bronchial dilator), for

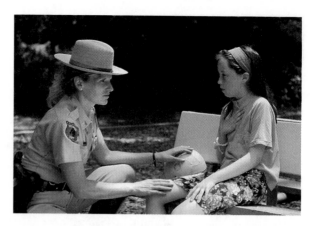

**Figure 5-1** Sitting can make breathing easier for victims in respiratory distress.

the condition if it is available. Continue to look and listen for any changes in the victim's vital signs. Help maintain normal body temperature by preventing chilling or overheating.

If the victim's breathing is rapid and you suspect that it is caused by emotion, such as excitement, try to calm the victim to slow the breathing. Reassurance is often enough to correct hyperventilation. You can also ask the victim to try to breathe with you. Breathe at a normal rate, emphasizing inhaling and exhaling.

If the condition does not improve, the victim may become unconscious. Keep the victim's airway open and monitor breathing. In many cases, hyperventilation caused by emotion will correct itself after the victim becomes unconscious.

## ◆ RESPIRATORY ARREST

Respiratory arrest is the condition in which breathing stops. It may be caused by illness, injury, or an obstructed airway. The causes of respiratory distress can also lead to respiratory arrest. In respiratory arrest the person gets no oxygen. The body can function for only a few minutes without oxygen before the body systems, especially the circulatory system, fail.

When the heart stops, other body systems will also start to fail. However, you can keep the person's respiratory system functioning artificially with rescue breathing.

## Rescue Breathing

**Rescue breathing** is a technique of breathing air into a person to supply the oxygen needed to survive. Rescue breathing works because the air you breathe into the victim contains more than enough oxygen to keep that person alive. The air you take in with every breath contains about 21 percent oxygen, but your body uses only a portion of that. The air you breathe out of your lungs and into the lungs of the victim contains about 16 percent oxygen, enough to keep someone alive.

Whenever possible, you should use breathing devices to provide rescue breathing. But since such devices are not always immediately available, you must also be able to perform rescue breathing without any airway adjuncts. In this chapter you will learn how to do rescue breathing. Chapter 6 covers the use of breathing devices during rescue breathing.

You will discover if you need to give rescue breathing during the first two steps of the ABCs in the primary survey, when you open the airway and check for breathing. If you cannot see, hear, or feel signs of breathing, give 2 slow breaths. Each breath should make the chest gently rise. Then check circulation by feeling for the pulse and looking for severe bleeding.

If the victim is not breathing but has a pulse, continue giving breaths. Remember to keep the airway open with the head-tilt/chin-lift (Fig. 5-2, *A*). The **head-tilt/chin-lift** not only opens the airway by moving the tongue away from the back of the throat but also moves the epiglottis from the opening of the trachea. Gently pinch the victim's nose shut with the thumb and index finger of your hand that is on the victim's forehead. Next, make a seal around the victim's mouth with your

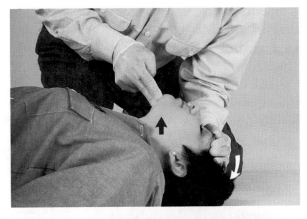

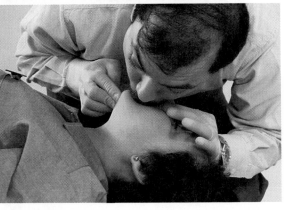

**Figure 5-2   A,** The head-tilt/chin-lift opens the victim's airway. **B,** To breathe for a nonbreathing victim, seal your mouth around the person's mouth and breathe slowly into the person.

mouth. Breathe slowly into the victim until you see the victim's chest rise (Fig. 5-2, *B*). Each breath should last about 1½ seconds, with a pause between breaths to let the air flow back out. Watch the victim's chest rise each time you breathe to make sure that your breaths are actually going in.

If you do not see the victim's chest rise and fall as you give breaths, you may not have the head tilted back far enough to open the airway adequately. Retilt the victim's head and try again to give breaths. If your breaths still do not go in, the victim's airway is obstructed. You must give the care for the obstructed airway that is described later in this chapter.

Check for a pulse after giving 2 slow breaths. If the victim has a pulse but is not breathing, continue rescue breathing by giving

1 breath every 5 seconds. A good way to time the breaths is to count, "one one-thousand, two one-thousand, three one-thousand." Then take a breath on four one-thousand and breathe into the victim on five one-thousand. Counting this way ensures that you give 1 breath about every 5 seconds.

After 1 minute of rescue breathing (about 12 breaths), recheck the pulse to make sure the heart is still beating. If the victim still has a pulse but is not breathing, continue rescue breathing. Check the pulse every minute. Do not stop rescue breathing unless one of the following occurs:

- The victim begins to breathe on his or her own.
- The victim has no pulse. Begin CPR (described in Chapter 7).
- Another rescuer with training equal to or greater than yours takes over for you.
- You are too exhausted to continue.

## ◆ SPECIAL CONSIDERATIONS FOR RESCUE BREATHING

### Air in the Stomach

When you do rescue breathing, air normally enters the victim's lungs. Sometimes, however, air may enter the victim's stomach for any of several reasons. First, breathing into the victim longer than about 1½ seconds may cause extra air to fill the stomach. Do not overinflate the lungs. Stop the breath when the chest has risen. Second, if the victim's head is not tilted back far enough, the airway will not open completely. As a result, the chest may only rise slightly. This will cause you to breathe more forcefully, causing air to enter the stomach. Last, breaths given too quickly create more pressure in the airway, causing air to enter the stomach. Slow breaths minimize pressure in the air passages.

Air in the stomach is called **gastric distention.** Gastric distention can be a serious problem because it can make the victim vomit. When an unconscious victim vomits, stomach

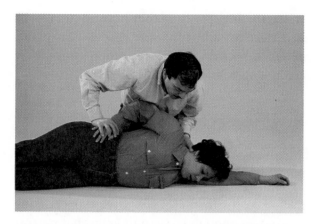

**Figure 5-3** If vomiting occurs, turn the victim on his or her side, and clear the mouth of any matter.

contents may get into the lungs, obstructing breathing. Taking such foreign material into the lungs is called **aspiration.** Aspiration can hamper your rescue breathing attempts.

### Vomiting

When you give rescue breathing, the victim may vomit whether or not there is gastric distention. If this happens, turn the victim's head and body together as a unit to the side (Fig. 5-3). This helps prevent vomit from entering the lungs. Quickly wipe the victim's mouth clean, carefully reposition the victim on his or her back, and continue with rescue breathing.

### Mouth-to-Nose Breathing

Sometimes you may not be able to make an adequate seal over a victim's mouth to perform rescue breathing. For example, the person's jaw or mouth may be injured or shut too tightly to open, or your mouth may be too small to cover the victim's. If so, provide mouth-to-nose rescue breathing as follows:

- Maintain the head-tilt position with one hand on the forehead. Use your other hand to close the victim's mouth, making sure to push on the chin, not on the throat.
- Open your mouth wide, take a deep breath, seal your mouth around the victim's nose,

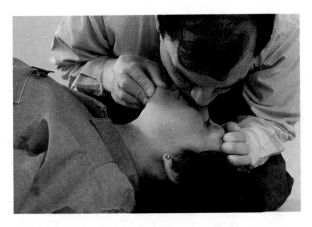

**Figure 5-4**  For mouth-to-nose breathing, close the victim's mouth, and seal your mouth around the victim's nose. Give slow breaths, watching the chest to see if the air goes in.

and breathe (Fig. 5-4). Open the victim's mouth between breaths, if possible, to let air escape.

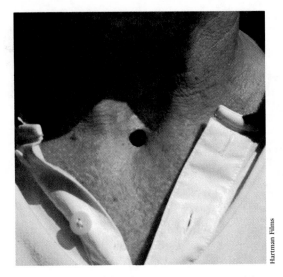

**Figure 5-5**  You may need to perform rescue breathing on a victim with a stoma.

## Mouth-to-Stoma Breathing

Some people have had an operation that removed all or part of the **larynx,** the upper end of the windpipe. They breathe through an opening called a **stoma** in the front of the neck (Fig. 5-5). Air passes directly into the trachea through the stoma instead of through the mouth and nose.

Most people with a stoma wear a medical alert bracelet or necklace or carry a card identifying this condition. You may not see the stoma immediately. You will probably notice the opening in the neck as you tilt the head back to check for breathing.

To give rescue breathing to someone with a stoma, you must give breaths through the stoma instead of the mouth or nose. Follow the same basic steps as in mouth-to-mouth breathing, except—

1. Look, listen, and feel for breathing with your ear over the stoma (Fig. 5-6, *A*).
2. Give breaths into the stoma, breathing at the same rate as for mouth-to-mouth breathing (Fig. 5-6, *B*).
3. Remove your mouth from the stoma between breaths to let air flow back out.

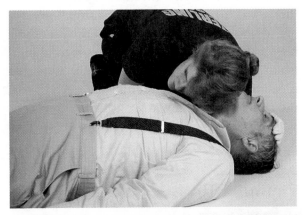

A

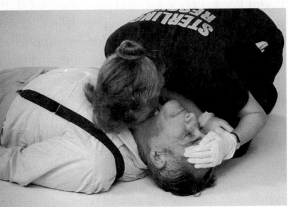

B

**Figure 5-6  A,** Look, listen, and feel for breathing with your ear over the stoma. **B,** Seal your mouth around the stoma and breathe into the victim. You may need to tilt the head back to get the chin out of the way.

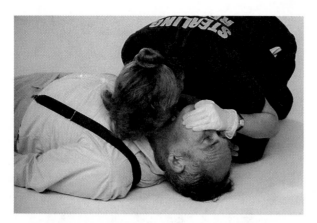

**Figure 5-7** When performing rescue breathing on a person with a stoma, you may need to seal the victim's nose and mouth to prevent air from escaping.

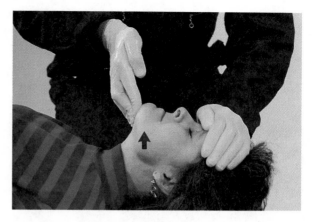

**Figure 5-8** If you suspect head or spine injuries, try to open the airway by lifting the chin without tilting the head.

If the chest does not rise when you give rescue breaths, suspect that the victim may have had only part of the larynx removed. That means that some air continues to flow through the larynx to the lungs during normal breathing. When giving mouth-to-stoma breathing, air may leak through the nose and mouth, diminishing the amount of your rescue breaths that reach the lungs. If this occurs, you need to seal the nose and mouth with your hand to prevent air from escaping during rescue breathing (Fig. 5-7).

## Victims with Dentures

If you know or see the victim is wearing **dentures,** do not automatically remove them. Dentures help rescue breathing by supporting the victim's mouth and cheeks during mouth-to-mouth breathing. If the dentures are loose, the head-tilt/chin-lift may help keep them in place. Remove the dentures only if they become so loose that they block the airway or make it difficult for you to give breaths.

## Suspected Head or Spine Injuries

You should suspect head or spine injuries in victims who have suffered a violent force, such as that caused by a motor vehicle crash, a fall, or a diving or other sports-related incident. If you suspect the victim may have an injury to the head or spine, you should try to minimize movement of the head and neck when opening the airway. This requires you to change the way you open the airway.

Try to open the victim's airway by lifting the chin without tilting the head back (Fig. 5-8). In most cases this will allow air to pass into the lungs. Since it is sometimes difficult to keep the jaw lifted with one hand, you can perform a two-handed jaw thrust technique (Fig. 5-9, *A*). Open the airway by placing your fingers under the angles of the jaw and lifting. Place your mouth over the victim's, using your cheek to close the nose, and breathe (Fig. 5-9, *B*). This technique allows you to open the airway and provide rescue breathing without moving the head.

## Infants and Children

Rescue breathing for infants and children follows the same general procedures as rescue breathing for adults. The minor differences take into account the infant's or child's undeveloped physique and moderately faster heartbeat and breathing rate. Rescue breathing for infants and children uses less air in each breath, and breaths are delivered at a slightly faster rate.

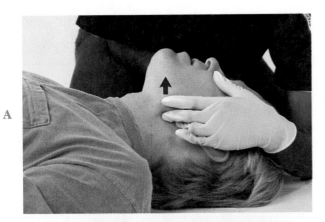

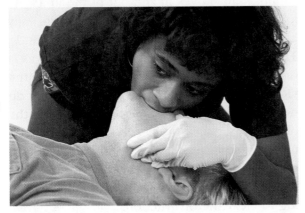

A

B

**Figure 5-9**  **A,** Use a two-handed jaw thrust when a chin-lift fails to open the airway of a victim with a suspected head or spine injury. **B,** Seal the nose with your cheek and breathe into the victim.

You do not need to tilt a child's or infant's head as far back as an adult's to open the airway. Tilt the head back only far enough to allow your breaths to go in. Tipping the head back too far in a child or infant may cause injury that will obstruct the airway. Give 1 slow breath every 3 seconds for a child or an infant. Figure 5-10 shows rescue breathing for an adult, a child, and an infant.

It is easier to cover both the mouth and nose of an infant with your mouth when giving breaths. Remember to breathe slowly into the victim. Each breath should last about 1½ seconds. Be careful not to overinflate a child's or infant's lungs. Breathe only until you see the chest rise. After 1 minute of rescue breathing (about 20 breaths in a child or an infant), recheck the pulse.

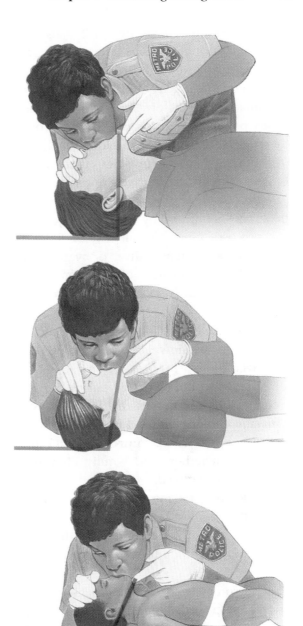

**Figure 5-10**  There are only minor differences in rescue breathing for adults, children, and infants.

## ◆ AIRWAY OBSTRUCTION

**Airway obstruction** is the most common cause of respiratory emergencies. The two types of airway obstruction are anatomical and mechanical.

An **anatomical obstruction** occurs when the airway is blocked by an anatomical structure such as the tongue or swollen tissues of the mouth and throat. This type of obstruction may result from injury to the neck or a medical emergency such as anaphylactic shock. The most common obstruction in an unconscious person is the tongue, which drops to the back of the throat and blocks the airway. This occurs because muscles, including the tongue, relax when deprived of oxygen.

A **mechanical obstruction** occurs when the airway is blocked by a foreign object, such as a piece of food, a small toy, or fluids like vomit, blood, mucus, saliva, or water. Someone with a mechanical obstruction may be choking. Common causes of choking include—

♦ Trying to swallow large pieces of poorly chewed food.
♦ Drinking alcohol before or during meals. Alcohol dulls the nerves that aid swallowing, making choking on food more likely.
♦ Wearing dentures. Dentures make it difficult to sense whether food is fully chewed before it is swallowed.
♦ Eating while talking excitedly or laughing, or eating too fast.
♦ Walking, playing, or running with food or objects in the mouth.

A person whose airway is blocked can quickly stop breathing, lose consciousness, and die. You must be able to recognize that the airway is obstructed and give care immediately. Because an obstructed airway is so serious, checking the airway comes first in the ABCs of the primary survey. If you mistake an obstructed airway for a heart attack or some other serious condition, you might be slow to provide the right kind of care or perhaps even give the wrong kind.

A person who is choking may have either a complete or partial airway obstruction. A victim with a **complete airway obstruction** is not able to breathe at all. With a partial airway obstruction, the victim's ability to breathe de-

pends on how much air can get past the obstruction into the lungs.

## Partial Airway Obstruction

A person with a **partial airway obstruction** can still move air to and from the lungs. This air allows the person to cough in an attempt to dislodge the object. The person may also be able to move air past the vocal cords to speak. The narrowed airway causes a wheezing sound as air moves in and out of the lungs. As a natural reaction to choking, the victim may clutch at the throat with one or both hands. This reaction is universally recognized as a distress signal for choking (Fig. 5-11). If the victim is coughing forcefully or wheezing, do not interfere with attempts to cough up the object. A person who has enough air to cough forcefully or speak also has enough air entering the lungs to breathe. Stay with the victim and encourage him or her to continue coughing to clear the obstruction.

## Complete Airway Obstruction

A partial airway obstruction can quickly become a complete airway obstruction. A person

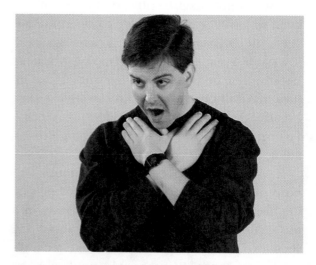

**Figure 5-11** Clutching the throat with one or both hands is universally recognized as a distress signal for choking.

with a completely blocked airway is unable to speak, cry, breathe, or cough effectively. Sometimes the victim may cough weakly and ineffectively or make high-pitched noises. All of these signs indicate the victim is not getting enough air to the lungs to sustain life. Act immediately.

## Care for Choking Victims

When someone is choking, you must try to reopen the airway as quickly as possible. Give **abdominal thrusts;** this technique is also called the **Heimlich maneuver.** Abdominal thrusts compress the abdomen, increasing pressure in the lungs and airway. This simu-

lates a cough, forcing trapped air in the lungs to push the object out of the airway like a cork from a bottle of champagne (Fig. 5-12).

## Care for a Conscious Choking Adult

To give abdominal thrusts to a conscious choking adult, stand behind the victim and wrap your arms around his or her waist (Fig. 5-13, *A*). The victim may be seated or standing. Make a fist with one hand and place the thumb side against the middle of the victim's abdomen just above the navel and well below the lower tip of the breastbone (Fig. 5-13, *B*). Grab your fist with your other hand and give quick upward thrusts into the abdomen (Fig. 5-13, *C*). Repeat these thrusts until the object

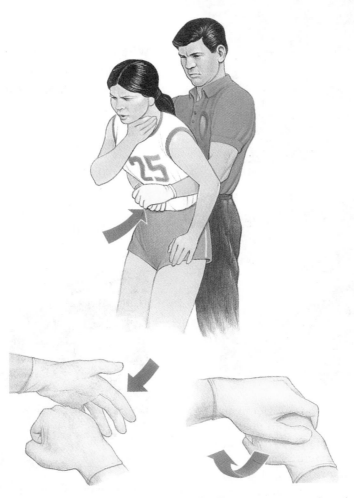

**Figure 5-12**  Abdominal thrusts simulate a cough, forcing air trapped in the lungs to push the object out of the airway.

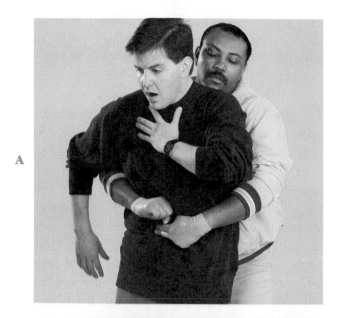

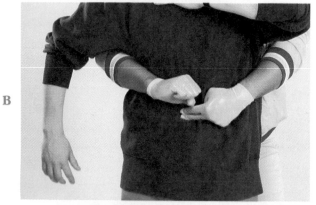

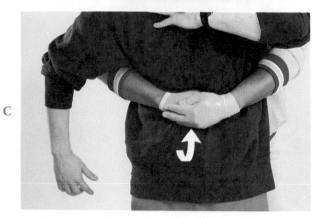

**Figure 5-13** **A,** Stand behind the victim and wrap your arms around his waist to give abdominal thrusts. **B,** Place the thumb side of your fist against the middle of the victim's abdomen. **C,** Grasp your fist with your other hand and give quick upward thrusts into the abdomen.

is dislodged or the victim becomes unconscious.

## If You Are Alone and Choking

If you are choking and no one is around who can help, you can give yourself abdominal thrusts in two ways: (1) Make a fist with one hand and place the thumb side on the middle of your abdomen slightly above your navel and well below the tip of your breastbone. Grasp your fist with your other hand and give a quick upward thrust. (2) You can also lean forward and press your abdomen over any firm object such as the back of a chair, a railing, or a sink (Fig. 5-14). Be careful not to lean over anything with a sharp edge or a corner that might injure you.

## Care for a Conscious Choking Adult Who Becomes Unconscious

When giving abdominal thrusts to a conscious choking victim, anticipate that the victim will become unconscious if the obstruction is not removed. If he or she becomes unconscious, lower the victim to the floor on his or her back. Take the following steps:

1. Open the airway by grasping the lower jaw and lifting the jaw up.
2. Attempt to dislodge and remove the object by sweeping it out with your index finger.

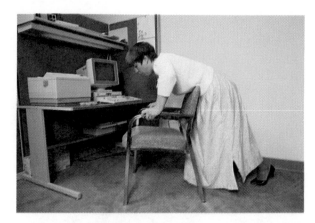

**Figure 5-14** To give yourself abdominal thrusts, press your abdomen onto a firm object, such as the back of a chair.

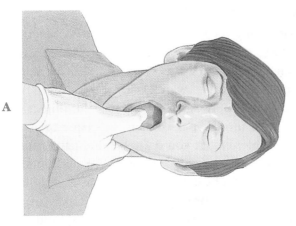

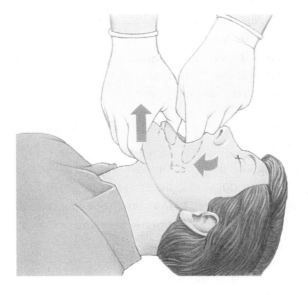

**Figure 5-15 A,** To do a finger sweep, first lift the lower jaw. **B,** Use a hooking action to sweep the object out of the airway.

This action is called a ***finger sweep*** (Fig. 5-15, *A-B*). When doing a finger sweep, use a hooking action to remove the object. Be careful not to push the object deeper into the victim's throat.

3. Try to open the victim's airway using the head-tilt/chin-lift.
4. Give 2 slow breaths. Often, the throat muscles relax enough after the person becomes unconscious to allow air past the obstruction and into the lungs.

If air does not go in,

5. Reposition (retilt) the head.
6. Give 2 slow breaths.

If air still does not go in, assume the airway is still obstructed.

7. Give up to 5 abdominal thrusts. To give abdominal thrusts to an unconscious victim, straddle one of the victim's thighs. Place the heel of one hand on the victim's abdomen, just above the navel and well below the lower tip of the breastbone. Place the other hand on top of the first. The fingers of both hands should point directly toward the victim's head (Fig. 5-16, *A-B*). Give quick upward thrusts into the abdomen.
8. Do a finger sweep.
9. Give 2 slow breaths. If the breaths do not go

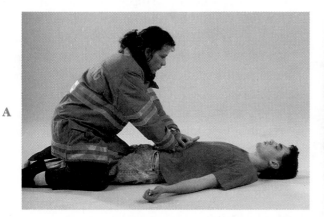

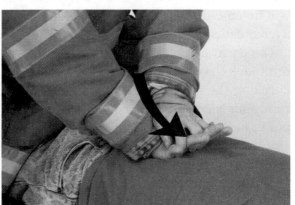

**Figure 5-16 A,** To give abdominal thrusts to an unconscious victim, straddle the victim's thighs. **B,** Position your hands with your fingers pointing toward the victim's head. Give quick, upward thrusts.

in, reposition the head and repeat 2 breaths. Repeat this sequence beginning with step 7 until the object is expelled, you can breathe air into the victim, or other trained personnel arrive and take over.

## Care for an Unconscious Choking Adult

During the primary survey, you may discover that an unconscious adult victim is not breathing and that the 2 slow breaths you give will not go in. If this happens, take the following steps:

1. Reposition the head.
2. Give 2 slow breaths again. You may not have tilted the victim's head back far enough the first time. If the breaths will not go in, assume the victim's airway is obstructed.
3. Give up to 5 abdominal thrusts.
4. Do a finger sweep.
5. Open the airway.
6. Give 2 slow breaths.

If breaths do not go in, go back to step 1 and repeat all steps until the object is dislodged, you can breathe air into the victim, or other trained personnel arrive and take over.

*If your first attempts to clear the airway are unsuccessful, do not stop.* The longer the victim goes without oxygen, the more the muscles will relax, making it more likely that you will be able to clear the airway enough to deliver breaths successfully.

Once you are able to breathe air into the victim's lungs, complete the initial assessment by checking the victim's pulse and checking and caring for any severe bleeding. If there is no pulse, begin CPR (see Chapter 7). If the victim has a pulse but is not breathing on his or her own, continue rescue breathing.

If the victim starts breathing on his or her own, monitor both breathing and pulse until more advanced medical personnel arrive and take over. Maintain an open airway; look, listen, and feel for breathing; and keep checking the pulse.

## When to Stop Thrusts

Stop giving thrusts immediately if the object is dislodged or if the person begins to breathe or cough. Make sure the object is cleared from the airway, and watch that the person is breathing freely again. Even after the object is coughed up, the person may still have breathing problems that you do not immediately see. You should also realize that both abdominal thrusts and chest thrusts may cause internal injuries. Therefore, any time thrusts are used to dislodge an object, the person should be taken to the nearest hospital emergency department for follow-up care, even if the victim seems to be breathing without difficulty.

# Special Considerations for Choking Victims

In some instances, abdominal thrusts are not the best method of care for choking victims. Some choking victims need chest thrusts. For example, if you cannot reach far enough around the victim to give effective abdominal thrusts, you should give chest thrusts. You should also give chest thrusts to pregnant choking victims.

## Chest Thrusts for a Conscious Victim

To give **chest thrusts** to a conscious victim, stand behind the victim and place your arms under the victim's armpits and around the chest. As you do for abdominal thrusts, make a fist with one hand, placing the thumb side against the center of the victim's breastbone. Be sure that the thumb is centered on the breastbone, not on the ribs. Also make sure that your fist is not near the lower tip of the breastbone. Grab your fist with your other hand and thrust inward (Fig. 5-17). Repeat these thrusts until the object is dislodged or the victim becomes unconscious.

## Chest Thrusts for an Unconscious Victim

With a pregnant, unconscious victim or any to whom you cannot effectively deliver abdomi-

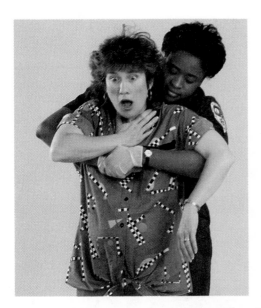

**Figure 5-17**  If you cannot reach around the victim to give abdominal thrusts or if the victim is noticeably pregnant, give chest thrusts.

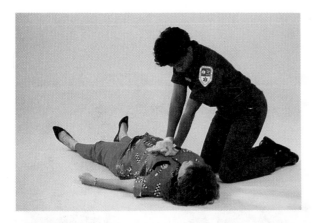

**Figure 5-18**  Positioning for Chest Thrusts for an Unconscious Victim

nal thrusts, give chest thrusts. Kneel next to the victim. Place the heel of one hand on the center of the victim's breastbone and your other hand on top of it (Fig. 5-18). Give up to 5 quick thrusts. Each thrust should compress the chest 1½ to 2 inches. After giving thrusts, do a finger sweep and give 2 slow breaths as you normally would for an unconscious choking victim. Repeat the sequence if the object is not expelled.

# Infants and Children

Choking emergencies are common in infants and children. Emergency care for a choking child is similar to the care for a choking adult. The only significant difference involves considering the child's size. Obviously, you cannot use the same force when giving abdominal thrusts to a child to expel the object. Care for infants who are choking includes a combination of chest thrusts given with two fingers and back blows given with the heel of one hand. Abdominal thrusts are not used for a choking infant because of their potential for causing injury.

## Care for a Conscious Choking Child

If you suspect that a child is choking, provide care as you would for an adult.

◆ Give abdominal thrusts. Stand or kneel behind the child. Wrap your arms around the child's waist. Make a fist with one hand. Place the thumb side of your fist against the middle of the child's abdomen just above the navel and well below the lower tip of the breastbone. Grasp your fist with your other hand and give quick, upward thrusts into the abdomen (Fig. 5-19, *A* and *B*).
◆ Repeat the thrusts until the obstruction is cleared or until the child becomes unconscious.

If the child coughs up the object or starts to breathe or cough, continue to watch the child to ensure that he or she is able to breathe normally. Even though the child may be breathing well, remember that he or she may have other problems that require a physician's attention.

## Care for an Unconscious Choking Child

If, during the primary survey, you determine that an unconscious child has a complete airway obstruction, continue care as follows:

1. Reposition the head.
2. Give 2 slow breaths again. You may not have

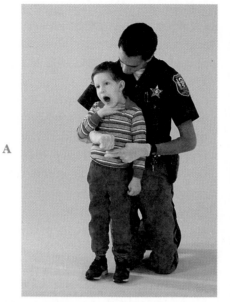

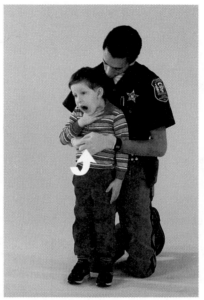

**Figure 5-19** To give abdominal thrusts to a child, **A,** stand or kneel behind the child. Wrap your arms around the child's waist. Make a fist with one hand. Place the thumb side of your fist against the middle of the child's abdomen, just above the navel and well below the tip of the breastbone. **B,** Grasp your fist with your other hand and give quick upward thrusts into the abdomen.

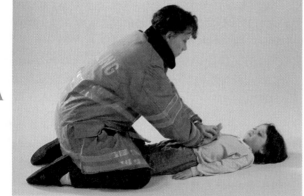

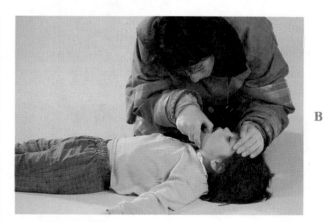

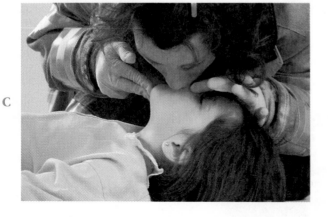

**Figure 5-20** To care for an unconscious child with a complete airway obstruction, **A,** give 5 abdominal thrusts. **B,** Do a finger sweep if you see the object. **C,** Open the airway and give 2 slow breaths.

tilted the child's head back far enough the first time. If the breaths will not go in, assume the child's airway is obstructed.

3. Give up to 5 abdominal thrusts.
4. Do a finger sweep if you see the object.
5. Open the airway.
6. Give 2 slow breaths (Fig. 5-20, *A, B,* and *C*).

If your breaths still do not go in, go back to step 1 and repeat all the steps until the obstruction is removed, the child starts to breathe or cough, or more advanced medical personnel arrive and take over.

## Care for a Conscious Choking Infant

If, during the primary survey, you determine that a conscious infant cannot breathe, cough, or cry, give care for a complete airway obstruction. Give 5 back blows followed by 5 chest thrusts.

Start by positioning the infant faceup on your forearm. Place your other arm on top of the infant, using your thumb and fingers to hold the infant's jaw while holding the infant securely between your forearms (Fig. 5-21, *A*). Turn the infant over so that he or she is facedown on your forearm (Fig. 5-21, *B*). Lower

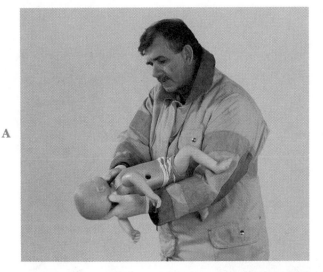
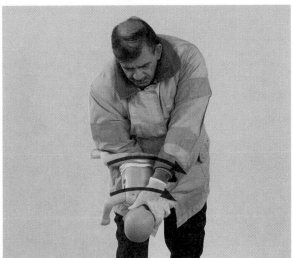
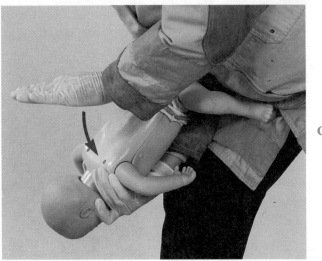

**Figure 5-21**  To give back blows, **A,** sandwich the infant between your forearms. Support the infant's head and neck by holding the jaw between your thumb and forefinger. **B,** Turn the infant over so that he or she is facedown on your forearm. **C,** Give 5 firm back blows with the heel of your hand while supporting the arm that is holding the infant on your thigh.

your arm onto your thigh so that the infant's head is lower than his or her chest. Give 5 firm back blows with the heel of your hand between the infant's shoulder blades (Fig. 5-21, *C*). Maintain support of the infant's head and neck by firmly holding the jaw between your thumb and forefinger.

To give chest thrusts, turn the infant back over. Start by placing your free hand and forearm along the infant's head and back so that the infant is held between your two hands and forearms. Continue to support the infant's head between your thumb and fingers from

the front while you cradle the back of the head with your other hand (Fig. 5-22, *A*).

Turn the infant onto his or her back. Lower your arm that is supporting the infant's back onto your thigh. The infant's head should be lower than his or her chest (Fig. 5-22, *B*). Give 5 chest thrusts (Fig. 5-22, *C*).

To locate the correct place to give chest thrusts, imagine a line running across the infant's chest between the nipples (Fig. 5-23, *A*). Place your ring finger on the breastbone just under this imaginary line. Then place the two fingers next to the ring finger just under the

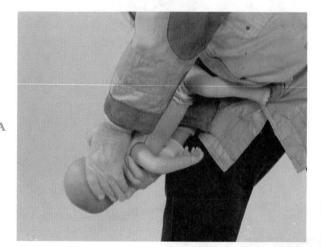
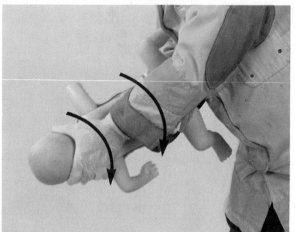
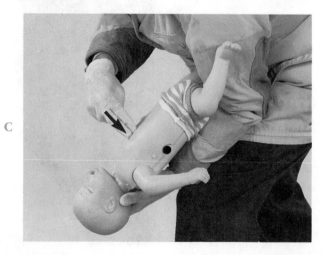

**Figure 5-22** To give chest thrusts, **A,** sandwich the infant between your forearms. Continue to support the infant's head. **B,** Turn the infant onto his or her back and support your arm on your thigh. The infant's head should be lower than the chest. **C,** Give 5 chest thrusts.

nipple line. Raise the ring finger (Fig. 5-23, *B*). If you feel the notch at the end of the infant's breastbone, move your fingers up a little bit.

Use the pads of the two fingers to compress the breastbone ½ to 1 inch, then let the breastbone return to its normal position. Keep your fingers in contact with the infant's breastbone. Compress 5 times. You can give back blows and chest thrusts effectively whether you stand up or sit. If the infant is large or your hands are too small to adequately support the infant, you may prefer to sit. Place the infant in your lap to give back blows and chest

thrusts. The infant's head should be lower than the chest (Fig. 5-24).

Keep giving back blows and chest thrusts until the object is coughed up or the infant begins to breathe or cough. Even if the infant seems to be breathing well, he or she should be examined by a physician.

## Care for an Unconscious Choking Infant

If, during the primary survey, you determine that an unconscious infant is not breathing and that the 2 slow breaths you give will not go in, position your hands and continue care as follows:

1. Reposition the head.
2. Give 2 slow breaths again. If the breaths will not go in, assume the infant's airway is obstructed.
3. Give 5 back blows.
4. Give 5 chest thrusts.
5. Do a foreign body check (see following).
6. Open the airway.
7. Give 2 slow breaths. If the breaths do not go in, go back to step 1 and repeat steps until the obstruction is removed, the infant starts to breath or cough, or more advanced medical personnel arrive and take over.

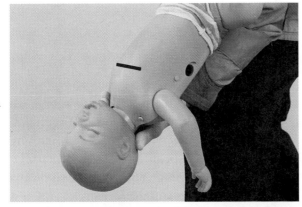
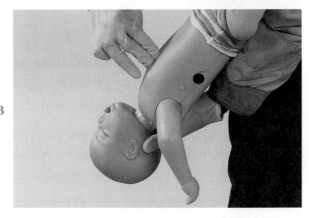

**Figure 5-23** To locate the correct place to give chest thrusts, **A,** imagine a line running across the infant's chest between the nipples. **B,** Place the pad of your ring finger on the breastbone just under this imaginary line. Place the pads of the 2 fingers next to the ring finger just under the nipple line. Raise the ring finger.

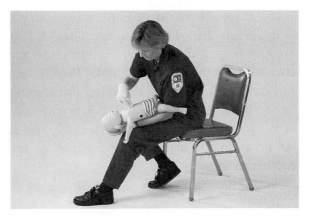

**Figure 5-24** If you cannot adequately support the infant, put him or her on your lap with the head lower than the chest.

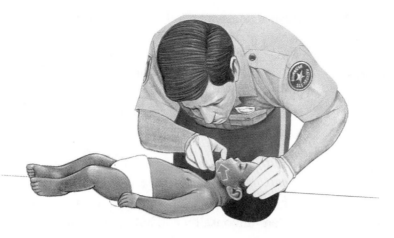
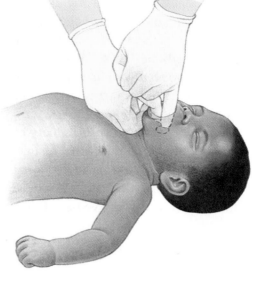
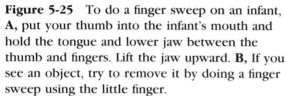

**Figure 5-25** To do a finger sweep on an infant, **A,** put your thumb into the infant's mouth and hold the tongue and lower jaw between the thumb and fingers. Lift the jaw upward. **B,** If you see an object, try to remove it by doing a finger sweep using the little finger.

To do a foreign body check—

- Stand or kneel beside the infant's head.
- Open the infant's mouth, using your hand that is nearer the infant's feet. Put your thumb into the infant's mouth and hold both the tongue and the lower jaw between the thumb and fingers. Lift the jaw upward (Fig. 5-25, *A*).
- Look for an object. If you can see it, try to remove it by doing a finger sweep with the little finger (Fig. 5-25, B).

If you are able to breathe air into the infant's lungs, finish the primary survey. Give 2 slow breaths as you did for rescue breathing, and check the infant's brachial pulse. Next, check and care for any severe bleeding. If the infant has no pulse, begin CPR, which you will learn in Chapter 7. If the infant has a pulse and is not breathing on his or her own, continue rescue breathing.

## ◆ SUMMARY

In this chapter you learned how to recognize and provide care for breathing emergencies. You know that you should look for a breathing emergency in the primary survey because it can be life-threatening. You learned the signs and symptoms of respiratory distress and respiratory arrest and the appropriate care for each condition. You also learned the basic techniques for rescue breathing and for special situations. Finally, you learned how to care for choking victims, both conscious and unconscious. By knowing how to care for breathing emergencies, you are now better prepared to care for other emergencies. You will learn about cardiac emergencies in the next chapter.

# ◆ Review Questions ◆

Circle the letter of the best answer.

**1.** When giving back blows to a choking infant, the head should be—
a. Higher than the chest.
b. Turned to the side.
c. Lower than the chest.
d. Resting on your thigh.

**2.** When performing rescue breathing, how often should you check to make sure the victim still has a pulse?
a. Every 5 minutes
b. Every minute
c. Every 10 minutes
d. Every 3 minutes

**3.** If you breathe too forcefully during rescue breathing, what will happen?
a. Air will go into the victim's stomach.
b. Oxygen will not get to the victim's tissues.
c. Air will not reach the victim's lungs.
d. The victim's pharynx will rupture.

**4.** When you provide rescue breathing to a victim, you are—
a. Artificially circulating oxygenated blood to the body cells.
b. Supplementing the air the victim is already breathing.
c. Supplying the victim with oxygen necessary for survival.
d. All of the above.

**5.** One sign of respiratory distress is—
a. Pain in the abdomen.
b. Rapid or slow breathing.
c. Constricted pupils.
d. Ringing in the ears.

**6.** Which is a common cause of choking?
a. Drinking alcohol before or during meals
b. Wearing dentures
c. Eating small pieces of well-chewed food
d. a and b

**7.** After discovering that the first 2 breaths are not causing the victim's chest to rise, what should you do?
a. Retilt the head and reattempt breaths.
b. Begin rescue breathing.
c. Breathe more forcefully.
d. Do a finger sweep.

**8.** Which would be included in your care for an unconscious choking child?
a. Positioning on the back
b. Repeated abdominal thrusts until the object is dislodged
c. Doing a foreign body check
d. a and c

**9.** When doing rescue breathing, breathe—
a. Forcefully, to make sure the air goes in.
b. Slowly, only until the chest gently rises.
c. Quickly, giving one breath every 2 seconds.
d. None of the above.

**Answers:** 1. c; 2. b; 3. a; 4. c; 5. b; 6. d; 7. a; 8. d; 9. b.

# Rescue Breathing for an Adult or a Child

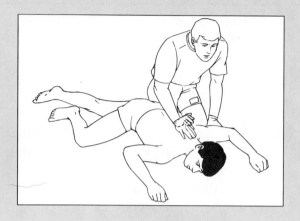

☐ **Check for consciousness**
- ◆ Tap or gently shake person.
- ◆ Shout, "Are you OK?"

**If person does not respond. . .**

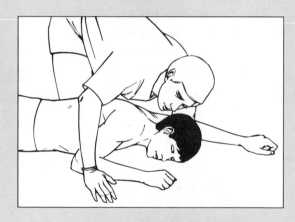

☐ **Check for breathing**
- ◆ Look, listen, and feel for about 5 seconds.

**If not breathing or you cannot tell. . .**

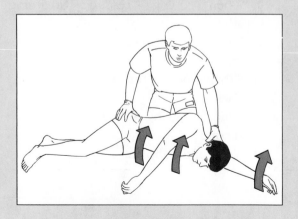

- ◆ Position victim on back. Roll person as a single unit while supporting the head and neck.

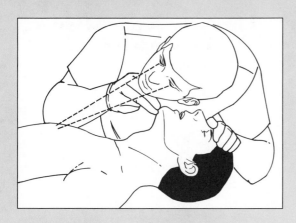

- ◆ Open the airway.
- ◆ Tilt head back and lift chin.
- ◆ Recheck breathing.
- ◆ Look, listen, and feel for about 5 seconds.

**If person is not breathing. . .**

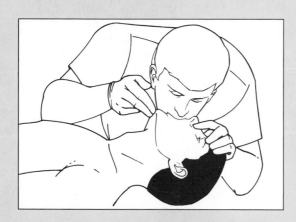

- ◆ Keep head tilted back.
- ◆ Pinch nose shut.
- ◆ Seal your lips tightly around person's mouth.
- ◆ Give 2 slow breaths, each lasting about 1½ seconds.
- ◆ Watch to see that the breaths go in.

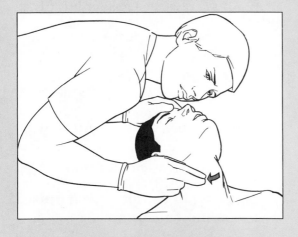

☐ **Check for a pulse**
- ◆ Locate Adam's apple.
- ◆ Slide fingers down into groove of neck on side closer to you.
- ◆ Feel for a pulse for 5 to 10 seconds.

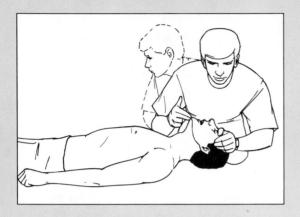

## ☐ Check for severe bleeding

- ♦ Look from head to toe for severe bleeding.

If person has a pulse and is not breathing. . .

- ♦ Do rescue breathing.

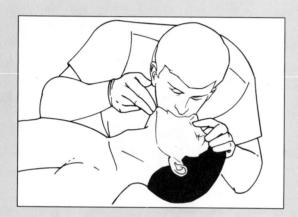

## ☐ Begin rescue breathing

- ♦ Maintain open airway with head-tilt/chin-lift.
- ♦ Pinch nose shut.
- ♦ Give 1 slow breath every 5 seconds (1 breath every 3 seconds for a child).
- ♦ Watch chest to see that your breaths go in.
- ♦ Continue for 1 minute—about 12 breaths (adult); about 20 breaths (child).

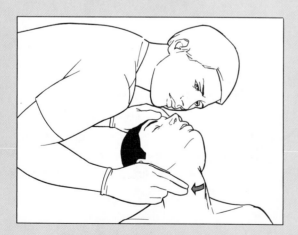

## ☐ Recheck pulse and breathing every minute

- ♦ Feel for pulse for about 5 seconds.
- ♦ Look, listen, and feel for breathing.

If person has a pulse and is breathing. . .

- ♦ Keep airway open.
- ♦ Monitor breathing.

If person has a pulse but is still not breathing. . .

- ♦ Continue rescue breathing.

If person does not have a pulse and is not breathing. . .

- ♦ Begin CPR.

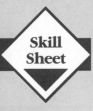

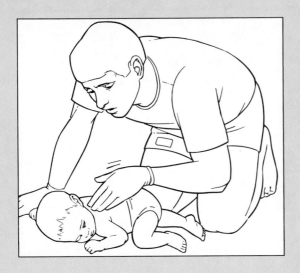

☐ **Check for consciousness**

♦ Tap or gently shake infant's shoulders.

If infant does not respond. . .

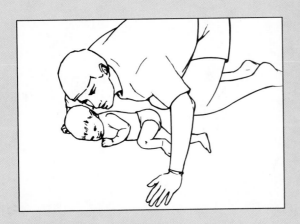

☐ **Check for breathing**

♦ Look, listen, and feel for about 5 seconds.

**If not breathing or you cannot tell. . .**

◆ Position infant on back. Roll infant onto back while supporting the head and neck.

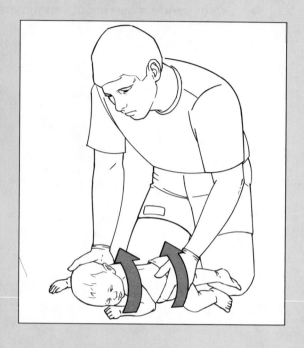

◆ Open the airway and recheck breathing.
◆ Tilt head back and lift chin.

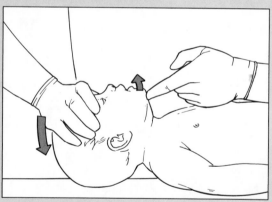

◆ Look, listen, and feel for about 5 seconds.

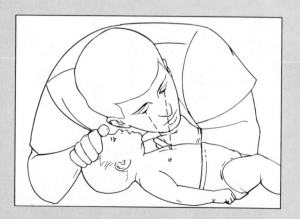

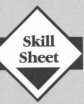
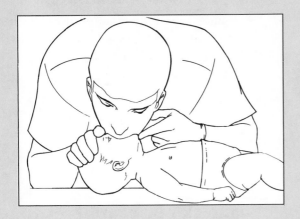

**If infant is not breathing. . .**

- ◆ Keep head tilted back.
- ◆ Seal your lips tightly around infant's mouth and nose.
- ◆ Give 2 slow breaths, each lasting about 1½ seconds.
- ◆ Watch to see that the breaths go in.

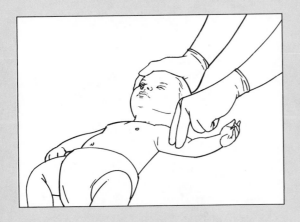

## ☐ Check for pulse

- ◆ Locate brachial pulse.
- ◆ Place fingers on the inside of upper arm, midway between elbow and shoulder.
- ◆ Feel for pulse for 5 to 10 seconds.

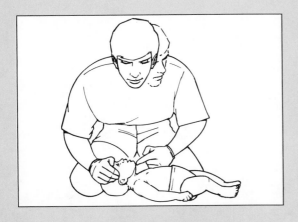

## ☐ Check for severe bleeding

- ◆ Look from head to toe for severe bleeding.

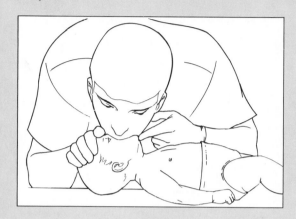

☐ **Begin rescue breathing**

- Maintain open airway with head-tilt/chin-lift.
- Give 1 slow breath every 3 seconds.
- Watch chest to see that your breaths go in.
- Continue for 1 minute—about 20 breaths.

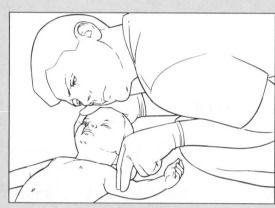

☐ **Recheck pulse and breathing every minute**

- Feel for pulse for about 5 seconds.
- Look, listen, and feel for breathing.

**If infant has a pulse and is breathing. . .**

- Keep airway open.
- Monitor breathing.

**If infant has a pulse but is still not breathing. . .**

- Continue rescue breathing.

**If infant does not have a pulse and is not breathing. . .**

- Begin CPR.

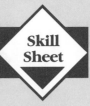
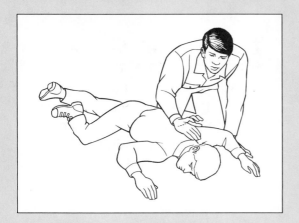

## ☐ Check for consciousness

- ♦ Tap or gently shake person.
- ♦ Shout, "Are you OK?"

**If person does not respond. . .**

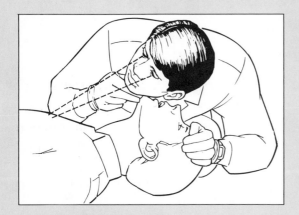

## ☐ Check for breathing

- ♦ Look, listen, and feel for breathing for about 5 seconds.

**If not breathing or you cannot tell. . .**

- ♦ Roll person as a single unit, while supporting the head and neck.
- ♦ Open the airway.
- ♦ Tilt head back and lift chin.
- ♦ Recheck breathing.
- ♦ Look, listen, and feel for about 5 seconds.

**If person is not breathing. . .**

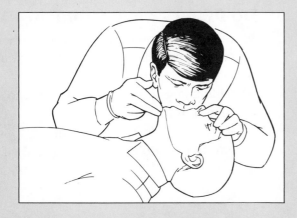

- ♦ Keep head tilted back.
- ♦ Pinch nose shut.
- ♦ Seal your lips tightly around person's mouth.
- ♦ Give 2 slow breaths, each lasting about 1½ seconds.
- ♦ Watch to see that the breaths go in.

If breaths do not go in. . .

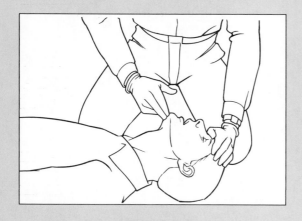

☐ **Retilt person's head and try 2 slow breaths again**

- ◆ Tilt person's head farther back.
- ◆ Pinch nose shut and seal your lips tightly around person's mouth.
- ◆ Give 2 slow breaths, each lasting about 1½ seconds.

If breaths still do not go in. . .

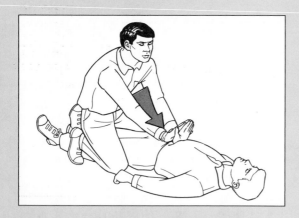

☐ **Give up to 5 abdominal thrusts**

- ◆ Place heel of 1 hand against middle of person's abdomen, just above the navel.
- ◆ Place other hand directly on top of first hand.
- ◆ Press into abdomen with upward thrusts.

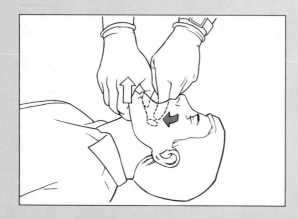

☐ **Do finger sweep (simulate)**

- ◆ Grasp both tongue and lower jaw between your thumb and fingers and lift jaw.
- ◆ Slide finger down inside of cheek to base of tongue.
- ◆ Attempt to sweep object out.
- ◆ For a child, do a finger sweep only if you see the object.

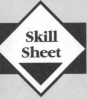
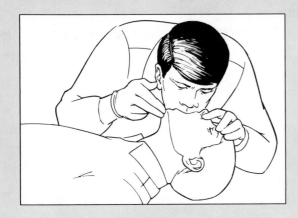

☐ **Open airway and give 2 slow breaths**

♦ Tilt head back.

♦ Pinch nose shut.

♦ Seal your lips tightly around person's mouth.

♦ Breaths should last about 1½ seconds.

♦ Watch chest to see if your breaths go in.

**If breaths still do not go in. . .**

♦ Retilt head and reattempt breaths.

♦ Continue with sequence of thrusts, finger sweeps, head tilt, 2 slow breaths, head retilt, and 2 slow breaths until. . .

    ◆ Obstruction is removed.

    ◆ Person starts to breathe or cough.

**If breaths go in. . .**

♦ Check pulse and breathing.

♦ If person has a pulse but is not breathing, do rescue breathing.

♦ If person does not have a pulse and is not breathing, do CPR.

♦ Check for and control severe bleeding.

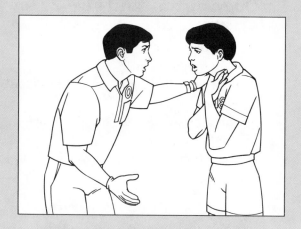

☐ **Determine whether person is choking**

♦ Ask, "Are you choking?"

**If person is choking. . .**

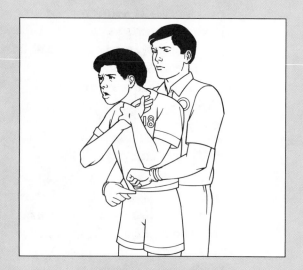

☐ **Give abdominal thrusts**

♦ Wrap your arms around person's waist.
♦ With one hand find the navel. With your other hand make a fist.
♦ Place thumb side of fist against middle of person's abdomen just above the navel and well below lower tip of breastbone.
♦ Grasp fist with your other hand.

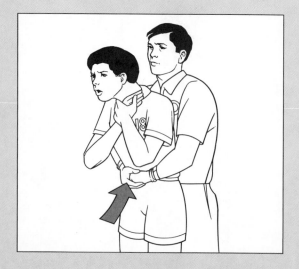

♦ Press fist into person's abdomen with a quick, upward thrust.
♦ Each thrust should be a separate and distinct attempt to dislodge the object.

**Repeat abdominal thrusts until. . .**

♦ **Object is coughed up.**
♦ **Person starts to breathe or cough forcefully.**
♦ **Person becomes unconscious.**
♦ **More advanced medical personnel arrive and take over.**

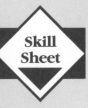
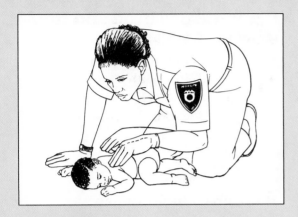

## ☐ Check for consciousness

♦ Tap or gently shake infant's shoulder.

*If infant does not respond. . .*

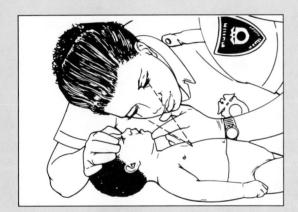

## ☐ Check for breathing

♦ Look, listen, and feel for about 5 seconds.

*If not breathing or you cannot tell. . .*

♦ Roll infant onto back while supporting the head and neck.
♦ Open the airway.
♦ Tilt head back and lift chin.
♦ Recheck breathing.
♦ Look, listen, and feel for about 5 sec-

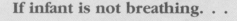

*If infant is not breathing. . .*

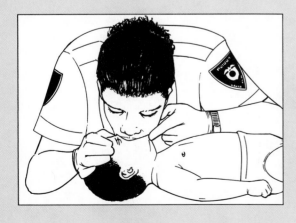

♦ Keep head tilted back.
♦ Seal your lips tightly around infant's mouth and nose.
♦ Give 2 slow breaths, each lasting about 1½ seconds.
♦ Watch to see that the breaths go in.

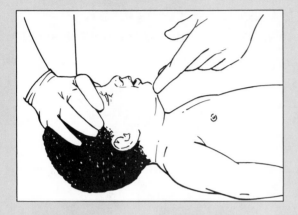

If breaths do not go in. . .

☐ **Retilt infant's head and try 2
slow breaths again**

- ◆ Tilt infant's head farther back.
- ◆ Seal your lips tightly around infant's
  mouth and nose.
- ◆ Give 2 slow breaths, each lasting
  about 1½ seconds.

If breaths still do not go in. . .

☐ **Give 5 back blows**

- ◆ Position infant facedown on forearm.
- ◆ Lower forearm onto thigh.
- ◆ Infant's head should be lower than
  feet.

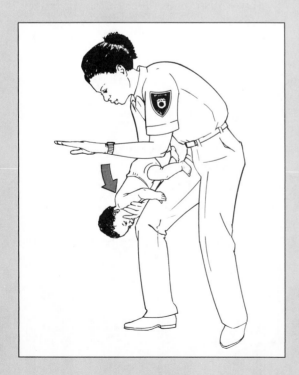

- ◆ Using the heel of your hand, give
  forceful back blows between infant's
  shoulder blades, 5 times.
- ◆ Each blow should be a separate and
  distinct attempt to dislodge the
  object.

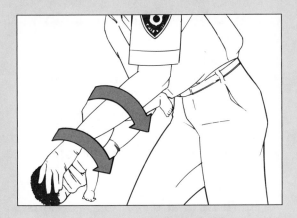

### ☐ Give 5 chest thrusts

- ◆ Position infant faceup on forearm.
- ◆ Lower forearm onto thigh.

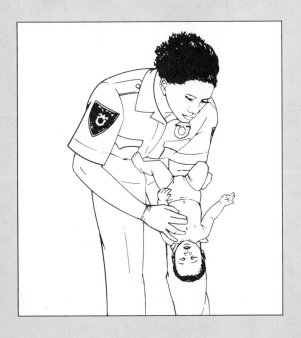

- ◆ Locate position for chest thrusts.
- ◆ Using pads of 2 fingers, smoothly compress breastbone ½ to 1 inch, 5 times.
- ◆ Each thrust should be a separate and distinct attempt to dislodge the object.

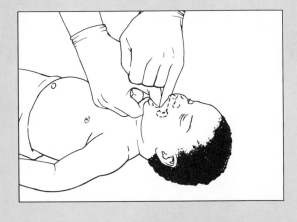

### ☐ Do foreign-body check

- ◆ Grasp both tongue and lower jaw between your thumb and fingers, and lift jaw.
- ◆ If object can be seen, slide little finger down inside of cheek to base of tongue.
- ◆ Attempt to sweep object out.

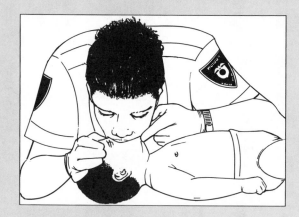

☐ **Open airway and give 2 slow breaths**

- ◆ Tilt head back.
- ◆ Seal your lips tightly around infant's mouth and nose.
- ◆ Give 2 slow breaths, each lasting about 1½ seconds.
- ◆ Watch to see if your breaths go in.

**If breaths still do not go in. . .**

- ◆ Retilt head and reattempt breaths.
- ◆ Continue with the sequence of back blows, chest thrusts, finger sweeps, head tilt, 2 slow breaths, head retilt, and 2 breaths until. . .
  - ◆ Obstruction is removed.
  - ◆ Infant starts to breathe, cry, or cough.
  - ◆ More advanced medical personnel arrive and take over.

**If breaths go in. . .**

- ◆ Check pulse and breathing.
- ◆ If infant has a pulse but is not breathing, do rescue breathing.
- ◆ If infant does not have a pulse and is not breathing, do CPR.
- ◆ Check and control severe bleeding.

◆ **Notes** ◆

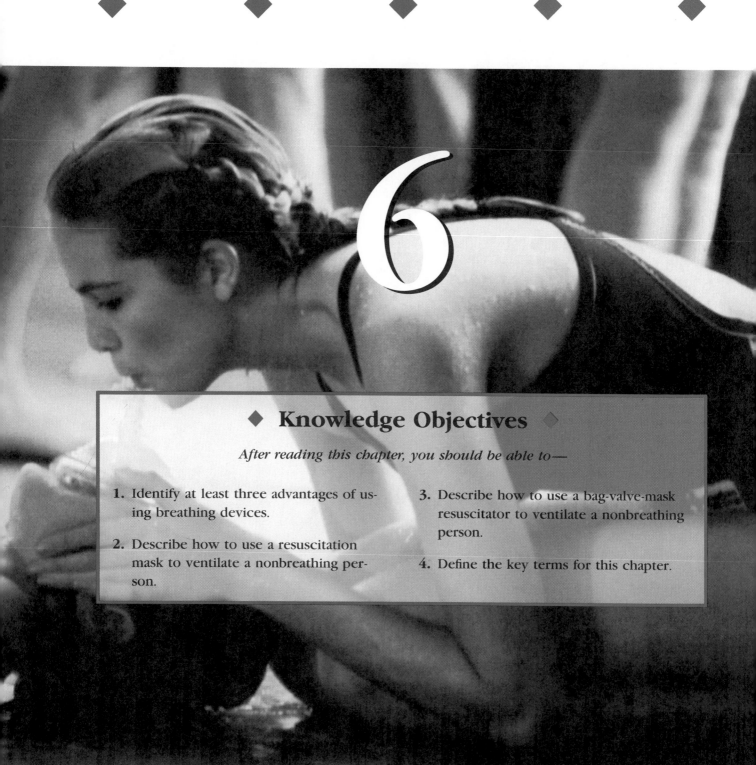

# Breathing Devices

**6**

◆ **Knowledge Objectives** ◆

*After reading this chapter, you should be able to—*

1. Identify at least three advantages of using breathing devices.

2. Describe how to use a resuscitation mask to ventilate a nonbreathing person.

3. Describe how to use a bag-valve-mask resuscitator to ventilate a nonbreathing person.

4. Define the key terms for this chapter.

## ◆ Skill Objectives ◆

*After reading this chapter and completing the course activities, you should be able to—*

1. Demonstrate on a manikin how to use a resuscitation mask to ventilate a non-breathing person.
2. Demonstrate on a manikin how to use a bag-valve-mask resuscitator to ventilate a nonbreathing person.
3. Make appropriate decisions about care when given an example of an emergency in which a person is not breathing.

## ◆ Key Terms ◆

**Bag-valve-mask (BVM) resuscitator:** A hand-held ventilation device, consisting of a self-inflating bag, a one-way valve, and a face mask; it can be used with or without supplemental oxygen.

**Breathing devices:** Devices used to help with ventilation.

**Resuscitation mask:** A pliable, dome-shaped device that fits over the nose and mouth, used to assist with rescue breathing.

**Ventilation:** The process of providing oxygen to the lungs through rescue breathing or by other means.

## ◆ Main Ideas ◆

1. The use of breathing devices can enhance your airway management skills.
2. The use of breathing devices such as a resuscitation mask or bag-valve mask help minimize the risk of disease transmission.
3. A resuscitation mask is a readily available and easily used device for ventilating a victim.
4. A bag-valve-mask resuscitator is most effective when used by two rescuers.

## ◆ INTRODUCTION

*A 45-year-old man who was experiencing chest pain is now unconscious, not breathing, and without a pulse.*

*A 60-year-old, unconscious woman has vomited and is not breathing. You know what must be done, but the sight of vomit causes you to hesitate. You overcome your reluctance, clean out her mouth, and begin rescue breathing.*

What do both of these situations have in common? Both are examples of situations in which **breathing devices,** used to help with ventilation, would have been desirable and could have enhanced the care you were providing. Breathing devices can contribute significantly to the survival and recovery of a seriously ill or injured person.

As you learned in previous chapters, airway management is critical in life-threatening situations. In this chapter you learn when and how to use two specific breathing devices to increase the effectiveness of the airway management you give a person who is injured or has suddenly become ill.

## ◆ BREATHING DEVICES

Many different breathing devices are commonly used in the prehospital setting. Which ones are routinely available to you will depend on your local standards and protocols. This chapter focuses on those breathing devices that you are likely to have immediately available or be asked to assist with in providing care. It is important to remember: *you should not delay care because a specific breathing device is not available.* Instead, you should start basic care, adding any breathing devices when they become available.

Breathing devices discussed in this chapter are resuscitation masks and bag-valve-mask resuscitators. In general, they provide several advantages. They can help you—

♦ Maintain an open airway.
♦ Perform rescue breathing.
♦ Limit the potential for disease transmission.
♦ Increase the oxygen concentration in a person's bloodstream.

## Resuscitation Masks

One of the most readily available, simple breathing devices for professional rescuers is the **resuscitation mask.** Resuscitation masks, such as the Laerdal Pocket Mask$_{TM}$, are pliable, dome-shaped devices that fit over a person's mouth and nose, aiding **ventilation** (providing oxygen to the lungs). Several types of resuscitation masks are available, varying in size, shape, and features (Fig. 6-1).

Resuscitation masks offer you several advantages. These include—

♦ Increasing the flow of air to the lungs by permitting air to travel through a person's mouth and nose at the same time.
♦ Providing an adequate seal for ventilation, even when a person has facial injuries.
♦ Providing an effective and easily accessible alternative to other methods of ventilation, such as mouth-to-mouth or mouth-to-nose breathing or bag-valve-mask resuscitation.
♦ Reducing the possibility of disease transmission by providing a barrier between the rescuer and the victim.

### Selecting a Resuscitation Mask

For a resuscitation mask to be most effective, it should meet the following criteria:

♦ Be made of a transparent, pliable material that allows you to make a tight seal on the person's face when you perform rescue breathing.

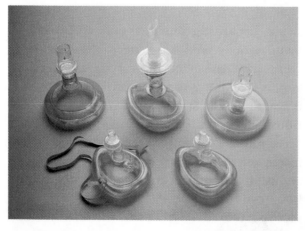

**Figure 6-1** Resuscitation masks vary in size, shape, and features.

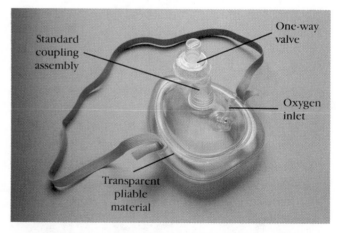

**Figure 6-2** A resuscitation mask should meet specific criteria.

# Supplemental Oxygen

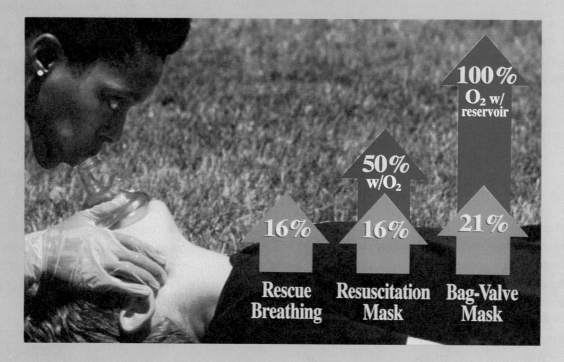

As you may recall, the normal concentration of oxygen in the blood is approximately 21 percent. Under normal conditions, this amount of oxygen is more than enough to sustain life. However, when serious injury or sudden illness occurs, the body does not function properly and can benefit from supplemental, or additional, oxygen. Without adequate oxygen, hypoxia will result. Hypoxia is a condition in which insufficient oxygen reaches the cells. When hypoxia occurs, it causes signs and symptoms that include increased breathing and heart rates, cyanosis, changes in consciousness, restlessness, and chest pain.

For example, a person having difficulty breathing and chest pain because of a heart attack or angina can have this pain and breathing discomfort reduced by the delivery of a higher concentration of oxygen. Supplemental oxygen delivered to the victim's lungs can help meet the increased demand for oxygen for all body tissues.

If a heart attack victim suddenly suffers cardiac arrest, then you must use rescue breathing to force air into the victim's lungs. Whether you perform rescue breathing using the mouth-to-mouth or mouth-to-mask method, the oxygen concentration you deliver to the victim is only 16 percent. This amount is adequate to sustain life in a healthy person. However, since chest compressions only circulate one-third normal blood flow under the best of conditions, body tissues are receiving only the bare minimum of oxygen required for short-term survival.

Using a bag-valve-mask resuscitator alone only improves the situation slightly, since it delivers atmospheric air (21 percent oxygen). A higher oxygen concentration helps to counter the effects of severe illness or injury to the body. Administering supplemental oxygen allows a substantially higher oxygen concentration, in some cases nearly 100 percent, to be delivered to the person.

◆ Have a one-way valve for releasing a person's exhaled air
◆ Have a standard 15 mm or 22 mm coupling assembly (the diameter of the opening that receives the one-way valve)
◆ Have an inlet for the delivery of supplemental oxygen
◆ Work well under a variety of environmental conditions such as extreme heat or cold
◆ Be easy to assemble and use

Figure 6-2 shows the features of an effective resuscitation mask.

## Using a Resuscitation Mask

Begin using a resuscitation mask by attaching the one-way valve to the mask. Next, position the mask so that it covers the person's mouth and nose. Place the wide end of the mask between the lower lip and chin. The narrow end of the mask should cover the nose. Figure 6-3, *A* and *B*, shows how to assemble and position a resuscitation mask.

When using a resuscitation mask, you must maintain a good seal to prevent air from leaking at the edges of the mask. Use both hands to hold the mask in place and to maintain an open airway. You do this by following three steps. They involve—

◆ Tilting the person's head back.
◆ Lifting the jaw upward.
◆ Keeping the person's mouth open.

Figure 6-4, *A* and *B* shows two methods for using a resuscitation mask.

If you suspect the victim has a head or spine injury, use the two-handed jaw thrust technique without head-tilt, described previously in Chapter 5. This technique can also be used with a resuscitation mask (Fig. 6-5). However, because the success of this technique depends on one's hand size and strength, some people will find it difficult to perform a two-handed jaw thrust using a resuscitation mask.

With the airway open and the mask sealed on the face, breathe slowly through the one-way valve, as you do for rescue breathing. Breathe only enough to make the chest gently rise.

## Bag-Valve-Mask Resuscitators

There are times when you will have a bag-valve-mask resuscitator available or be asked to assist with one. A **bag-valve-mask (BVM) resuscitator** is a hand-held device, like the resuscitation mask, used primarily to ventilate a

A 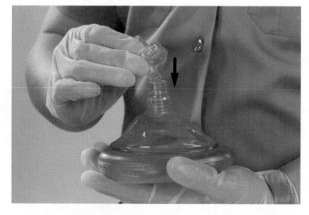 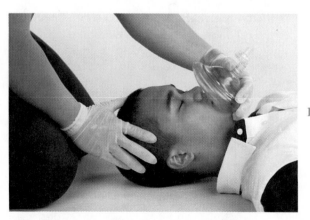 B

**Figure 6-3**  To use a resuscitation mask, **A,** attach the one-way valve to the mask. **B,** Position the mask to cover the mouth and nose.

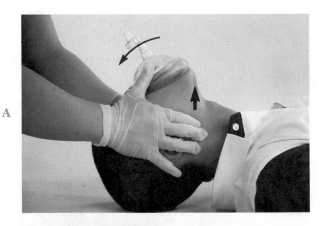

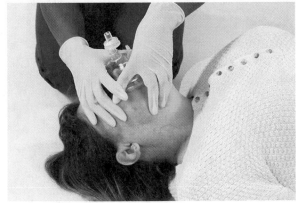

**Figure 6-4 A,** Use three steps to maintain an open airway and hold a resuscitation mask in place. **B,** Holding the mask from the side is an alternative method for using a resuscitation mask, for example, during one-person CPR.

nonbreathing person but also used to assist ventilation of a person who is in respiratory distress.

The device has three main components: bag, valve, and mask (Fig. 6-6). The bag is self-inflating. Once compressed, it reinflates automatically. The one-way valve allows air to move from the bag to the victim but prevents the victim's exhaled air from entering the bag. The mask is similar to a resuscitation mask.

The principle of the BVM is simple. By placing the mask on the victim's face and squeezing the bag, you open the one-way valve, forcing air into the victim's lungs. When you release the bag, the valve closes and air from the atmosphere or an oxygen cylinder refills the bag. At approximately the same time, the victim exhales. This exhaled air is diverted into the atmosphere through the closed one-way valve.

## Using a Bag-Valve-Mask Resuscitator

In the hands of a well-practiced rescuer, the bag-valve-mask resuscitator is effective. However, studies have shown that without consistent practice, single rescuers have a difficult time maintaining a tight enough seal and also maintaining an open airway for effective ventilation. For this reason, it is best if a BVM is used by two rescuers when possible.

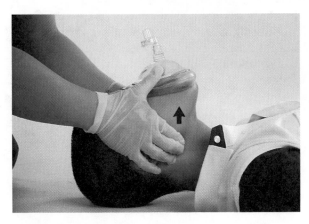

**Figure 6-5** When you suspect a head or spine injury, use the two-handed jaw thrust with a resuscitation mask.

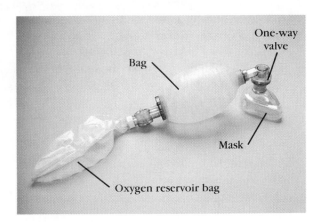

**Figure 6-6** A bag-valve-mask (BVM) resuscitator consists of a bag, valve, and mask.

# Oxygen-Powered Resuscitators: The Controversy Continues

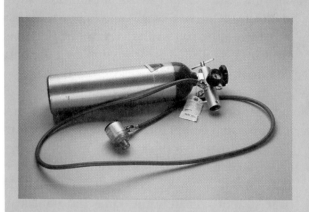

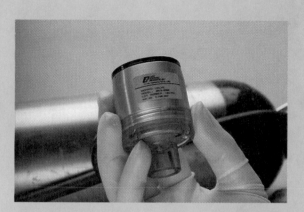

Oxygen-powered resuscitators, commonly called demand valves, have been the subject of controversy for several years. The points of controversy are whether these devices are as easy to use and whether they are as safe as other oxygen delivery devices. As the name "demand valve" implies, the victim can get oxygen on demand automatically.

A demand valve works in much the same way as a bag-valve-mask (BVM) resuscitator. However, instead of using a self-inflating bag as the ventilation source, it uses pressurized oxygen. The demand valve consists of a mask, a one-way valve, and an oxygen source. The mask is basically the same as that of the BVM unit. The one-way valve is designed to open and allow oxygen to flow to the breathing victim upon inhalation. The rescuer must depress a button to force oxygen into the lungs of a nonbreathing person. The use of the demand valve to ventilate a nonbreathing person is commonly called positive pressure resuscitation.

There are both advantages and disadvantages to using a demand valve. Advantages include delivery of a high concentration of oxygen (approaching 100 percent), ease of use, and protection from disease transmission. Also, like the resuscitation mask and BVM, the demand valve can deliver oxygen to either breathing or nonbreathing victims.

The disadvantages include higher cost compared with other devices, requirement of a constant source of oxygen, and rapid depletion of a cylinder. In addition, because the oxygen is delivered under higher pressure, complications from overventilation have been reported. This resulted in manufacturers designing demand valves that restricted oxygen flow and installing relief valves to eliminate overinflation when ventilating nonbreathing victims. However, this created another problem. This new restricted-flow demand valve did not always meet the needs of a person in severe respiratory distress. In addition, even with these restrictions, the device should not be used to ventilate nonbreathing children or infants because of the possibility that the device will overinflate the victim.

Some EMS systems have stopped using demand valves. Others use both the newer restricted demand valve for nonbreathing victims and the traditional demand valve for breathing victims. At the present, manufacturers are working to produce one demand valve more appropriate for both breathing and nonbreathing victims.

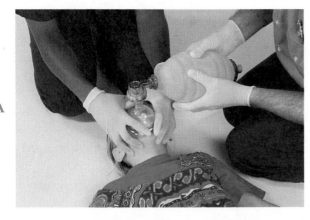
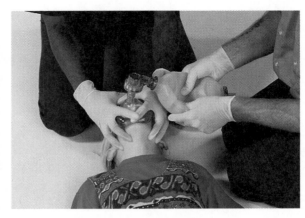

**Figure 6-7**  When two rescuers are available, **A,** one holds the mask in position and maintains an open airway, while **B,** the other ventilates the victim.

When two rescuers are using a BVM, one rescuer positions the mask and opens the victim's airway. This is done in the same way as previously described for resuscitation masks. While the first rescuer maintains a tight seal with the mask on the victim's face, the second rescuer provides ventilation by squeezing the bag until the victim's chest rises (Fig. 6-7, *A* and *B*). The bag should always be squeezed smoothly, not forcefully. This two-person technique is preferred because one rescuer can maintain an open airway and a tight mask seal while a second rescuer can provide ventilation.

### Advantages and Disadvantages

Using the bag-valve-mask resuscitator has distinct advantages and disadvantages.

Advantages:

* It delivers a higher concentration of oxygen than that delivered during mouth-to-mouth or mouth-to-mask rescue breathing.
* It limits the potential for disease transmission.
* It is very effective when used by two rescuers.

Disadvantages:

* It is not an easy one-person skill to master.
* Without regular practice, staying proficient is difficult.
* Assembly may take longer than other breathing devices.
* It is not readily available to all professional rescuers.

### ◆ SUMMARY

Although they are not required, breathing devices, such as resuscitation masks, can make the emergency care you provide safer, easier, and more effective. The resuscitation mask and BVM are the most appropriate devices for professional rescuers. They can significantly increase the oxygen concentration that an ill or injured person needs, help ventilate a non-breathing person, and reduce the likelihood of disease transmission.

These devices are appropriate for almost all types of injury or illness in which breathing may be impaired. Knowing how to use these devices will enable you to provide more effective care until more advanced medical care arrives.

# ◆ **Review Questions** ◆

**1.** Advantages of using breathing devices include—
a. Reducing the possibility of disease transmission.
b. Helping to perform rescue breathing.
c. Reducing the amount of oxygen in a victim's bloodstream.
d. a and b.

**2.** A resuscitation mask—
a. Permits air to flow through a person's nose and mouth at the same time.
b. Cannot be used when a person has facial injuries.
c. Cannot be used with supplemental oxygen.
d. All of the above.

**3.** When using a resuscitation mask, you—
a. Place the mask so it covers the victim's mouth and nose.
b. Tilt the victim's head back and lift the jaw.
c. Keep the victim's mouth open.
d. All of the above.

**4.** How does a bag-valve mask differ from a resuscitation mask?
a. It does not help prevent disease transmission.
b. It is usually more effective when used by two rescuers.
c. It can be used for victims in respiratory arrest.
d. All of the above.

**5.** Which is a disadvantage of the bag-valve mask?
a. It does not form a tight seal on a victim's face.
b. It takes regular practice to stay proficient.
c. It is not readily available to all professional rescuers.
d. b and c.

**Answers** 1. d; 2. a; 3. d; 4. b; 5. d.

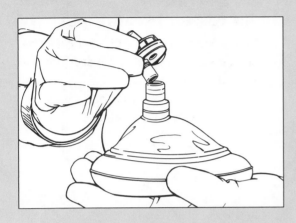

## ☐ Assemble the mask

- ◆ Attach one-way valve to mask.

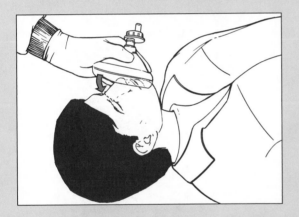

## ☐ Position the mask

- ◆ Kneel behind person's head.
- ◆ Place rim of mask between lower lip and chin.
- ◆ Cover victim's mouth and nose with mask.

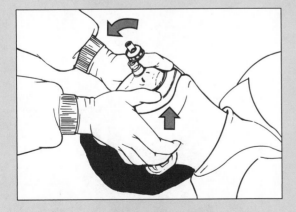

## ☐ Seal mask and open airway

- ◆ Place your thumbs on each side of mask to hold it in place.
- ◆ Place fingers of both hands along victim's jawbone.
- ◆ Tilt the head back.
- ◆ Apply downward pressure with thumbs while lifting the jaw upward with fingers.

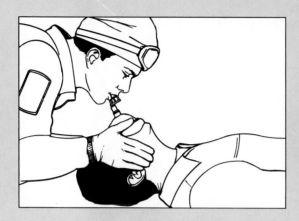

☐ **Begin rescue breathing**

♦ Give 1 slow breath about every 5 seconds (once about every 3 seconds for a child or infant).

♦ Watch chest to see that breaths go in.

♦ Recheck pulse every minute.

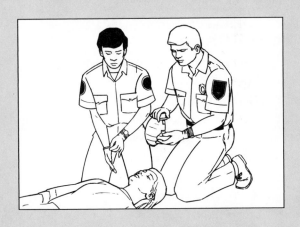

☐ **First rescuer—Assemble the BVM**

- ◆ Attach bag and valve to mask.

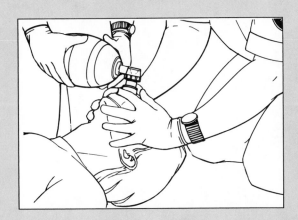

☐ **Position the mask**

- ◆ Place mask so that it covers victim's mouth and nose.

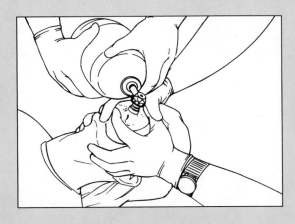

☐ **Seal mask and open airway**

- ◆ Place your thumbs on each side of mask to hold it in place.
- ◆ Place fingers of both hands along victim's jawbone.
- ◆ Tilt head back.
- ◆ Apply downward pressure with thumbs while lifting jaw upward with fingers.

**113**

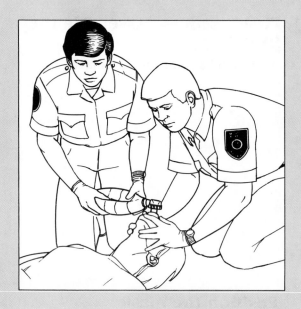

☐ **Second rescuer—Begin ventilations**

- ◆ Squeeze bag smoothly until victim's chest rises.
- ◆ Give 1 ventilation about every 5 seconds (once about every 3 seconds for a child or infant).
- ◆ Watch chest to see that ventilations go in.
- ◆ Recheck pulse every minute.

# ◆ Notes ◆

# Cardiac Emergencies

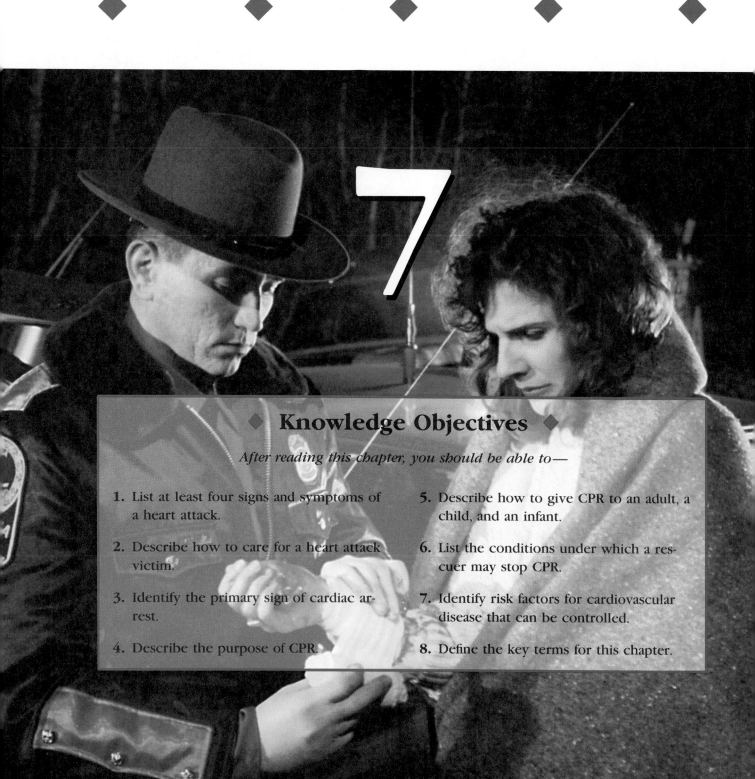

◆ **Knowledge Objectives** ◆

*After reading this chapter, you should be able to—*

1. List at least four signs and symptoms of a heart attack.

2. Describe how to care for a heart attack victim.

3. Identify the primary sign of cardiac arrest.

4. Describe the purpose of CPR.

5. Describe how to give CPR to an adult, a child, and an infant.

6. List the conditions under which a rescuer may stop CPR.

7. Identify risk factors for cardiovascular disease that can be controlled.

8. Define the key terms for this chapter.

# ◆ Skill Objectives ◆

*After reading this chapter and completing the class activities, you should be able to—*

1. Demonstrate how to give CPR to an adult, a child, and an infant.

2. Make appropriate decisions about care when given an example of an emergency in which a person is in cardiac arrest.

# ◆ Key Terms ◆

Cardiac arrest: A condition in which the heart has stopped or beats too irregularly or too weakly to pump blood effectively.

Cardiac emergencies: Sudden illnesses involving the heart.

Cardiopulmonary resuscitation (CPR): A technique that combines rescue breathing and chest compressions for a victim whose breathing and heart have stopped.

Cardiovascular disease: A disease of the heart and blood vessels; commonly known as heart disease.

Cholesterol: A fatty substance made by the body and found in certain foods.

Coronary arteries: Blood vessels that supply the heart muscle with oxygen-rich blood.

Heart: A fist-sized, muscular organ that pumps blood throughout the body.

Heart attack: A sudden illness involving the death of heart muscle tissue when it does not receive enough oxygen-rich blood.

Risk factors: Conditions or behaviors that increase the chance that a person will develop a disease.

# ◆ Main Ideas ◆

1. The most prominent symptom of a heart attack is persistent chest pain or discomfort. Most people who die from a heart attack die within 1 to 2 hours after the first signs and symptoms occur.

2. The absence of a pulse is the primary sign of cardiac arrest. The victim needs cardiopulmonary resuscitation (CPR). CPR artificially takes over the functions of the heart and lungs.

3. The cardiac arrest victim needs immediate CPR combined with early defibrillation and other advanced care for survival.

4. Most cardiac emergencies in infants and children are preventable.

5. CPR for infants and children is similar to CPR for adults. Techniques are modified because of smaller body size and faster breathing and heart rates.

6. In two-rescuer CPR, rescuers share the responsibility for performing rescue breathing and chest compressions.

7. The conditions that lead to heart attack build up over a number of years. Heart attacks and heart disease can be prevented.

## ♦ INTRODUCTION

In the primary survey you identify and care for immediate threats to a victim's life. Your priorities are to care for the victim's airway, breathing, and circulation (the ABCs). In Chapter 4 you learned how to open a victim's airway and assess breathing. In Chapter 5 you learned how to provide rescue breathing for a victim who has a pulse but is not breathing.

In this chapter you will learn how to recognize and provide care for **cardiac emergencies,** sudden illnesses involving the heart. You will learn the care for a victim with persistent chest pain and for one whose heart stops beating. The condition in which the heart stops, known as **cardiac arrest,** sometimes results from a heart attack. To provide care for a cardiac arrest victim, you need to learn how to perform CPR. Properly performed, CPR can keep a victim's vital organs supplied with oxygen-rich blood until more highly trained personnel arrive to provide advanced care.

This chapter also identifies the important risk factors for cardiovascular disease. It is as important to prevent heart attacks and cardiac arrests as it is to learn how to recognize them when they occur and provide appropriate care. Learn to modify your behavior to prevent cardiovascular disease in yourself.

## ♦ HEART ATTACK

The heart is protected by the ribs and sternum in front and by the spine in back (Fig. 7-1). It has four chambers and is separated into right and left halves. Oxygen-poor blood enters the right side of the heart and is circulated to the lungs, where it picks up oxygen. The now oxygen-rich blood returns to the left side of the heart, where it is circulated to all parts of the body. One-way valves direct the flow of blood as it moves through each of the heart's four chambers (Fig. 7-2). For the circulatory sys-

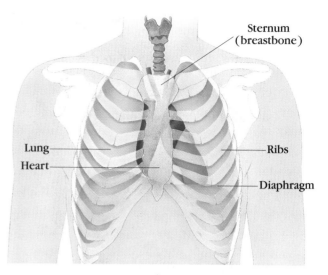

**Figure 7-1** The heart is located in the middle of the chest, behind the lower half of the sternum.

tem to be effective, the respiratory system must also be working so that the blood can pick up oxygen in the lungs.

As you read in Chapter 2, the cells of the heart need a continuous supply of oxygen-rich blood. If heart muscle tissue is deprived of oxygen-rich blood, it dies, and the victim may have a **heart attack.** A heart attack interrupts the heart's electrical system. This may result in an irregular heartbeat, which prevents blood from circulating effectively.

## Common Causes of Heart Attack

Heart attack is usually the result of cardiovascular disease. **Cardiovascular disease**—disease of the heart and blood vessels—is the leading cause of death for adults in the United States. It is estimated that approximately 66 million Americans have some form of cardiovascular disease. Each year nearly 1 million deaths are attributed to cardiovascular disease. Of these, more than 500,000 result from heart attacks, and most of them are sudden deaths.

Cardiovascular disease develops slowly. Deposits of **cholesterol,** a fatty substance made by the body, and other material may gradually

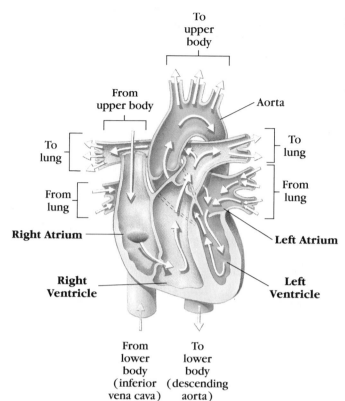

To
upper
body

From
upper body

Aorta

To
lung

To
lung

From
lung

From
lung

**Right Atrium**

**Left Atrium**

**Right
Ventricle**

**Left
Ventricle**

From
lower
body
(inferior
vena cava)

To
lower
body
(descending
aorta)

**Figure 7-2** The heart has four chambers and is separated into right and left halves. The right side receives blood from the body and sends it to the lungs. The left side receives blood from the lungs and circulates it out through the body. One-way valves direct the flow of blood through the heart.

= Oxygen-poor blood circulated from the body to the lungs

= Oxygen-rich blood circulated from the lungs to the body

build up on the inner walls of the arteries. This buildup results in a progressive narrowing of the arteries, a condition called **atherosclerosis.** Narrowing of the coronary arteries is a common form of coronary artery disease. When the coronary arteries narrow, a heart attack may occur (Fig. 7-3, *A* and *B*). Atherosclerosis can also involve arteries in other parts of the body, such as the brain. Diseased arteries in the brain can lead to **stroke,** a disruption of blood flow to a part of the brain.

Because atherosclerosis develops gradually, it can go undetected for many years. Even with significantly reduced blood flow to the heart muscle, there may be no signs and symptoms of heart trouble. Most people with atherosclerosis are unaware of it. As the narrowing progresses, some people experience symptoms such as chest pain. This is an early warning sign that the heart is not receiving enough oxygen-rich blood. Others may suffer a heart attack or even cardiac arrest without any pre-

## How the Heart Functions

Too often we take our hearts for granted. The heart is extremely reliable. The heart beats about 70 times each minute, or more than 100,000 times a day. During the average lifetime, the heart will beat nearly 3 billion times. The heart moves about a gallon of blood per minute through the body. This is about 40 million gallons in an average lifetime. The heart moves blood through about 60,000 miles of blood vessels.

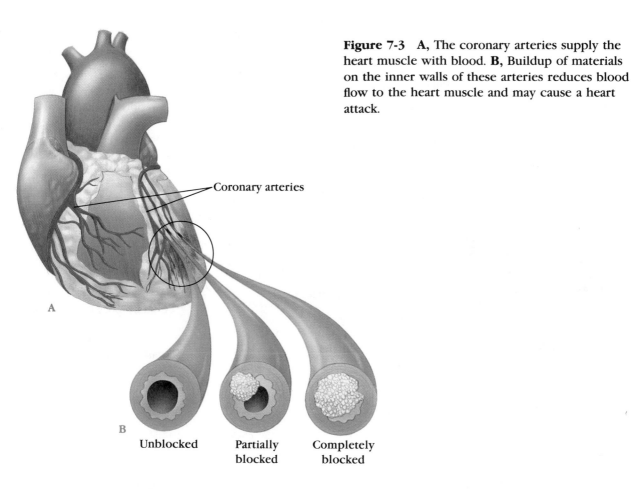

**Figure 7-3 A,** The coronary arteries supply the heart muscle with blood. **B,** Buildup of materials on the inner walls of these arteries reduces blood flow to the heart muscle and may cause a heart attack.

Coronary arteries

A

B

Unblocked

Partially blocked

Completely blocked

## The Brain Makes a Comeback

Neuroscientists have been mystified for years by the capricious effects of stroke. For many stroke survivors, talking becomes a tangle of words, a word like "piddlypop" spilling out in place of "hello." One man spoke normally unless he was asked to name fruits and vegetables. Each stroke survivor seemed to have a unique, perplexing set of problems, and doctors found recovery equally unpredictable.

But research into brain function after a stroke has shed new light on the way the brain works. Many strokes are caused when blood flow to the brain is cut off by a blood clot or hemorrhage. The oxygen-deprived brain cells rupture and die. Neuroscientists once believed that the cells died from lack of oxygen. However, their conclusion did not explain why stroke survivors sometimes get worse over several hours.

The oxygen-deprived brain cells actually start an avalanche of death when they rupture. The ruptured cells release huge quantities of the amino acid glutamate that gushes into surviving brain cells and destroys them. Normally, small amounts of glutamate act as transmitters between the cells, but large amounts are extremely damaging. Researchers believe that if they could inhibit the reaction of glutamate within the cell, they could stop the avalanche.

Researchers are developing several drugs to try to block the amino acid avalanche after a stroke. Oddly enough, they have found that drugs similar to phencyclidine, a potent animal tranquilizer and street drug known as PCP, have proven the most effective. Like PCP, the drugs cause temporary hallucinations. But doctors say the promising results outweigh the side effects.

Strokes still present many mysteries, but with more than 2 million people surviving strokes in the United States, doctors are hopeful that the drugs will eventually eliminate the long-term effects.

vious warning. Fortunately, this process can be slowed or stopped by lifestyle changes, such as forming healthy eating habits. Later in this chapter, you will learn ways to promote a lifestyle that is healthy for your heart.

## Signs and Symptoms of a Heart Attack

The most prominent symptom of a heart attack is persistent chest pain or discomfort. However, it may not always be easy for you to distinguish between the pain of a heart attack and chest pain caused by indigestion, muscle spasms, or other conditions. Brief, stabbing chest pain or pain that feels more intense when the victim bends or breathes deeply is usually not caused by a heart attack.

The pain of a heart attack can range from mild discomfort to an unbearable crushing sensation in the chest. The victim may describe it as an uncomfortable pressure, squeezing, tightness, aching, constricting, or heavy sensation in the chest. Often the victim feels pain in the center of the chest behind the sternum. It may spread to the shoulder, arm, neck, or jaw (Fig. 7-4). The pain is constant and usually not relieved by resting, changing position, or taking oral medication. Any chest pain that is severe, lasts longer than 10 minutes, or is accompanied by other heart attack signs and symptoms should receive emergency medical care immediately.

Although a heart attack is often dramatic, heart attack victims can have relatively mild initial symptoms. The victim can often mistake the symptoms for indigestion or gas. Some heart attack victims feel no chest pain or discomfort.

Some people with coronary artery disease may have chest pain or pressure that comes and goes and is not generally caused by a heart attack. This type of pain is called **angina pectoris.** Angina pectoris develops when the heart needs more oxygen-rich blood than it gets, such as during physical activity or emo-

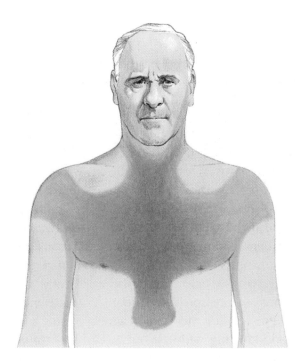

**Figure 7-4** Heart attack pain is most often felt in the center of the chest, behind the sternum. It may spread to the shoulder, arm, neck, or jaw.

tional stress. This lack of oxygen can cause a constricting chest pain that may spread to the neck, jaw, and arms.

Pain associated with angina usually lasts less than 10 minutes. A victim who knows he or she has angina will often have a prescribed medication to help relieve the pain. Reducing the heart's demand for oxygen, such as by stopping physical activity and by taking prescribed medication, often relieves angina. Administering oxygen to victims having angina helps relieve chest pain.

Another sign of a heart attack is difficulty breathing. The victim may be breathing faster than normal because the body is trying to get much-needed oxygen to the heart. Depending on the victim's general condition, the pulse may be faster or slower than normal or irregular. The victim's skin may be pale or bluish, particularly around the face. The skin may also be moist from perspiration. Some heart attack victims sweat profusely. These signs result from the stress the body experiences when the heart does not work effectively.

Since any heart attack may lead to cardiac arrest, it is important to recognize and act on these signs and symptoms. Prompt action may prevent cardiac arrest. A heart attack victim whose heart is still beating has a far better chance of living than a victim whose heart has stopped. Most people who die from a heart attack do so within 1 to 2 hours after the first signs and symptoms appear. Many could be saved if the victim or bystanders are aware of the signs and symptoms of a heart attack and act promptly. Victims often do not realize they are having a heart attack because they may dismiss the symptoms as indigestion or muscle soreness. Since most heart attacks result from blood clotting within arteries, early treatment of an attack with medication that dissolves clots has been helpful in minimizing damage to the heart.

Remember, the key symptom of a heart attack is persistent chest pain. If the victim states that chest pain is severe or chest discomfort has been present for more than 10 minutes, begin to care for the victim immediately.

## Care for a Heart Attack

The most important step in providing care is to recognize that any of the signs and symptoms listed in Table 7-1 may be those of a heart attack. You must take immediate action if any of these appear. A heart attack victim will probably deny the seriousness of the symptoms he or she is experiencing. Do not let this influence you. If you think there is a possibility that a person is having a heart attack, you must act. Have the victim stop what he or she is doing and rest comfortably. Many heart attack victims find it easier to breathe while sitting (Fig. 7-5).

Continue with your secondary survey. Talk to bystanders and the victim, if possible, to get more information. If the victim is having persistent chest pain, ask the following:

♦ When did the pain start?
♦ What brought it on?
♦ Does anything lessen it?
♦ What does it feel like?
♦ Where does it hurt?

Ask the victim if he or she has a history of heart disease. Some people who have heart disease have prescribed medications for chest pain. A medication often prescribed for angina is nitroglycerin, a small tablet that is dissolved under the tongue. Sometimes a nitroglycerin patch is placed on the chest. Once absorbed into the body, nitroglycerin enlarges the blood vessels to make it easier for blood to reach heart muscle tissue. The pain is relieved because the heart does not have to work so

### Table 7-1  Signs and Symptoms of a Heart Attack

| Signs and Symptoms | Characteristics |
| --- | --- |
| Persistent chest pain or discomfort | Persistent pain or pressure in the chest that is not relieved by resting, changing position, or oral medication<br>Pain may range from discomfort to an unbearable crushing sensation<br>Pain may radiate to the shoulders, arms, neck, or back |
| Breathing difficulty | Victim's breathing is noisy<br>Victim feels short of breath<br>Victim breathes faster than normal |
| Changes in pulse rate | Pulse may be faster or slower than normal or may be irregular |
| Skin appearance | Victim's skin may be pale or bluish in color<br>Victim's face may be moist, or victim may sweat profusely |

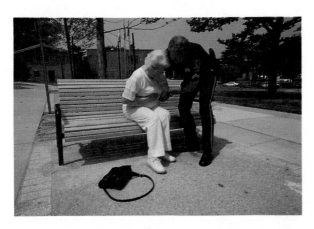

**Figure 7-5** The heart attack victim should rest in a position that helps breathing.

hard and oxygen delivery to the heart is increased.

Administer oxygen if it is available and you are trained to do so. Surviving a heart attack often depends on how soon the victim receives **advanced cardiac life support (ACLS),** the use of special equipment to maintain breathing and circulation for the victim of a cardiac emergency.

Be calm and reassuring when caring for a heart attack victim. Comforting the victim helps reduce anxiety and eases some of the discomfort. Continue to monitor the vital signs. Watch for any changes in appearance or behavior. Since the heart attack may cause cardiac arrest, be prepared to give CPR.

## ◆ CARDIAC ARREST

### What Is Cardiac Arrest?

Cardiac arrest occurs when the heart stops beating or beats too irregularly or too weakly to circulate blood effectively. Without a heartbeat, breathing soon stops. The condition when the heart stops beating and breathing stops is referred to as **clinical death.** Cardiac arrest is a life-threatening emergency because the vital organs of the body are no longer receiving oxygen-rich blood. Every year more than 300,000 heart attack victims die of cardiac arrest before reaching a hospital.

## Common Causes of Cardiac Arrest

Cardiovascular disease is the most common cause of cardiac arrest. Other causes include drowning, suffocation, certain drugs, severe injuries to the chest, severe loss of blood, and electrocution. Stroke and other types of brain damage can also stop the heart.

## Signs of Cardiac Arrest

A victim in cardiac arrest is not breathing and does not have a pulse. The victim's heart has either stopped beating or is beating so weakly or irregularly that it cannot produce a pulse. The absence of a pulse is the primary sign of cardiac arrest. No matter how hard you try, you will not be able to feel a pulse. If you cannot feel a carotid pulse, no blood is reaching the brain. The victim will be unconscious and breathing will stop.

Although cardiac arrest can result from a heart attack, cardiac arrest can also occur suddenly and independent of a heart attack. Therefore, the victim may not have shown the signs and symptoms of a heart attack before the cardiac arrest. This is called **sudden death.**

## Care for Cardiac Arrest

A victim who is not breathing and has no pulse is clinically dead. However, the cells of the brain and other vital organs will continue to live for a few minutes until the oxygen in the bloodstream is depleted. This victim needs **cardiopulmonary resuscitation (CPR).** The term *cardio* refers to the heart, and *pulmonary* refers to the lungs. CPR is a combination of rescue breathing and chest compressions. These chest compressions make the blood circulate when the heart is not beating. Given together, rescue breathing and chest compressions artificially take over the functions of the lungs and heart.

CPR increases a cardiac arrest victim's chances of survival by keeping the brain sup-

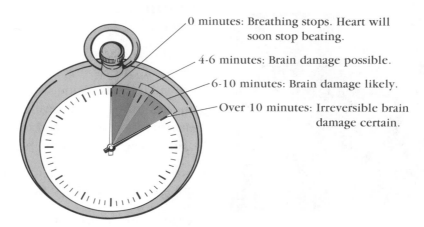

0 minutes: Breathing stops. Heart will soon stop beating.

4-6 minutes: Brain damage possible.

6-10 minutes: Brain damage likely.

Over 10 minutes: Irreversible brain damage certain.

**Figure 7-6** Clinical death is a condition in which the heart and breathing stop. Without resuscitation, clinical death will result in biological death. Biological death is the irreversible death of brain cells.

plied with oxygen until the victim receives advanced medical care. Without CPR, the brain will begin to die within 4 to 6 minutes. The irreversible damage caused by brain cell death is known as **biological death** (Fig. 7-6). Be aware that, at best, CPR only generates about one third of the normal blood flow to the brain.

CPR alone is not enough to help someone survive cardiac arrest. Advanced medical care is needed immediately. Trained emergency personnel can provide advanced cardiac life support (ACLS). Acting as an extension of a hospital emergency department, EMTs and paramedics can administer medications or use a defibrillator as part of their emergency care (Fig. 7-7).

A **defibrillator** is a device that sends an electric shock through the chest to the heart to start the heart beating effectively again. **Defibrillation** given as soon as possible is the key to helping some victims survive cardiac arrest. The time from collapse to defibrillation is critical. Immediate CPR must be combined with early defibrillation and other forms of ACLS to give the victim of cardiac arrest the best chance for survival.

Now commonplace, new defibrillators called **automatic external defibrillators (AEDs)** are part of the EMS system's emer-

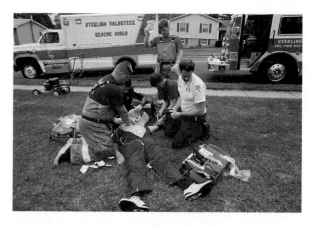

**Figure 7-7** Use of a defibrillator and other advanced measures may restore a heartbeat in a victim of cardiac arrest.

gency equipment. Today, AEDs are available for use by trained individuals in factories, stadiums, and other places where large numbers gather. Soon, automatic defibrillators may be used even more commonly. (Appendix A is an instructional unit on AEDs.)

In all cases of cardiac arrest, it is very important to start CPR promptly and continue it until a defibrillator is available. When a defibrillator is not available, CPR should be continued. Effective rescue breathing and chest compressions can help keep the brain, heart, and other vital organs supplied with oxygen-rich blood. Any delay in starting CPR or unnecessary delay in continuing it reduces the victim's chance for survival.

It might help to know that even in the best of situations, when CPR is started promptly, victims of cardiac arrest do not often survive. Controlling your emotions and accepting death are not easy. Remember that any attempt to resuscitate is worthwhile. Since performing CPR and defibrillation are not the only factors that determine whether a cardiac arrest victim survives, you should feel assured that you did everything you could to help.

## ♦ CPR FOR ADULTS

### Chest Compressions

It is not entirely understood why giving CPR circulates blood. The theory most widely held today is that chest compressions create pressure within the chest cavity that moves blood through the circulatory system. For compressions to be most effective, the victim should be face up on a firm, flat surface. The victim's head should be on the same level as the heart or lower. CPR is much less effective if the victim is on a soft surface, such as a sofa or mattress, or is sitting up in a chair.

### Finding the Correct Hand Position

Using the correct hand position, which is over the lower half of the **sternum** (breastbone), allows you to give the most effective compressions and minimize injury. At the lowest point of the sternum is an arrow-shaped piece of hard tissue called the **xiphoid.** You should avoid pressing directly on the xiphoid, which can break and injure underlying tissues.

To locate the correct hand position for chest compressions, find the lower edge of the victim's rib cage. Slide your middle and index fingers up the edge of the rib cage to the notch where the ribs meet the sternum (Fig. 7-8, *A*). Place your middle finger on this notch. Position your index finger next to your middle finger. Place the heel of your other

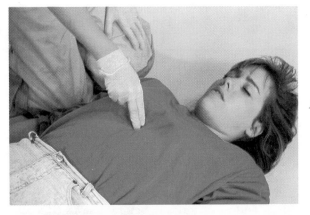

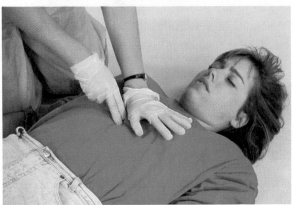

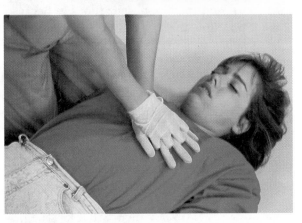

**Figure 7-8** **A,** Find the notch where the lower ribs meet the sternum. **B,** Place the heel of your hand on the sternum, next to your index finger. **C,** Place your other hand over the heel of the first hand. Use the heel of your bottom hand to apply pressure on the sternum.

hand on the sternum next to your index finger (Fig. 7-8, *B*). The heel of your hand should rest along the length of the sternum.

Once the heel of your hand is in position on the sternum, place your other hand di-

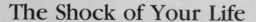

# The Shock of Your Life

Every year, 300,000 to 400,000 Americans collapse in cardiac arrest in their homes and on the streets. Ninety-five percent will not survive, but the development of a simple, computerized electric-shocking device offers an opportunity to increase survival.

In two thirds of all cardiac arrests, the heartbeat flutters chaotically before it stops, a condition called ventricular fibrillation. The electrical impulses that cause the heart muscle to function are no longer synchronized and fail to create the strong action needed to circulate the blood.

Electric-shocking devices, or defibrillators, were introduced onto mobile coronary units in 1966.[1] The machines allowed emergency personnel to monitor the heart's electrical rhythm. A doctor attached electrodes to the victim and reviewed the heart's rhythm. If necessary, an electric shock was delivered to the heart to try to restore its proper rhythm. Paramedics eventually took the place of doctors in evaluating rhythms and administering shocks. Because there were too few trained personnel across the United States, cardiac arrest victims were not always able to get the lifesaving help they needed.

Fortunately, a new, easy-to-use Automatic External Defibrillator (AED) allows emergency medical technicians, first responders, and even citizen responders to provide the lifesaving shocks. With the new defibrillators, a computer chip, rather than an advanced medical professional, analyzes the heart's rhythm. Typically, the first responder places the two electrodes on the victim's chest and then presses two buttons—first "ANALYZE," then "SHOCK." The machine does the rest.

AEDs monitor the heart's electrical activity through two electrodes placed on the chest. On a heart monitor, ventricular fibrillation looks like a chaotic, wavy line, whereas a normal heartbeat shows a pattern of evenly spaced, well-defined spiked points. The computer chip determines the need for a shock by looking at the pattern, size, and frequency of the electrocardiogram waves.

If the rhythm resembles ventricular fibrillation, the machine readies an electrical charge. When the electrical charge disrupts the irregular heartbeat, it is called defibrillation. This allows the heart's natural electrical system to begin to fire off electrical impulses correctly so the heart can beat normally.

When first responders are trained to use AEDs, they can drastically reduce the amount of time it takes to administer a shock in a cardiac emergency, researchers say. By extending training to first responders, communities increase the numbers of emergency personnel trained to use AEDs. In Eugene and Springfield, Oregon, AEDs were placed on every firetruck, and all fire fighters were trained to use them. Researchers saw these communities' survival rates for cardiac arrest increase by 18 percent in the first year.[2]

Most states recognize defibrillator training for EMTs. AEDs also are being introduced in areas that hold large groups of people, such as convention centers, stadiums, large businesses, and industrial complexes. Some health experts hope that someday AEDs will be as commonplace as fire alarms.

rectly on top of it (Fig. 7-8, *C*). Use the heel of your hand to apply pressure on the sternum. Try to keep your fingers off the chest by interlacing them or holding them upward. Applying pressure with your fingers can cause inefficient chest compressions or unnecessary damage to the chest. Positioning the hands correctly provides the most effective compressions. It also decreases the chance of pushing the xiphoid into the delicate organs beneath it, although this rarely occurs.

If you have arthritis or a similar condition in your hands or wrists, you may use an alternative hand position. Find the correct hand

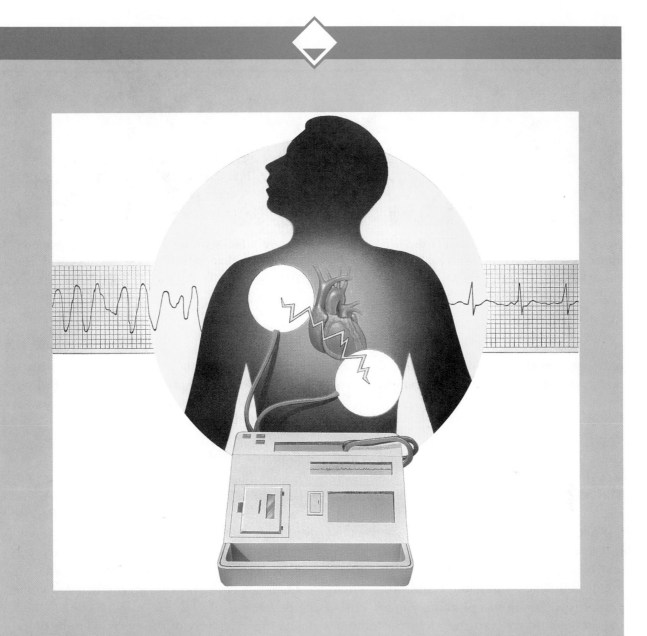

**REFERENCES**

1. Pantridge JF, Geddes JS: A mobile intensive care unit in the treatment of myocardial infarction, *Lancet* 2:271, 1967.

2. Graves JR, Austin D Jr, Cummins RO: *Rapid zap: automated defibrillation,* Englewood Cliffs, NJ, 1989, Prentice-Hall.

position in the same way, then grasp the wrist of the hand on the chest with your other hand (Fig. 7-9).

The victim's clothing will not necessarily interfere with your ability to position your hands correctly. If you can find the correct position without removing thin clothing, such as a T-shirt, do so. Sometimes a layer of thin clothing will help keep your hands from slipping, since the victim's chest may be moist with sweat. However, if you are not sure that you can find the correct hand position, bare the victim's chest. You should not be overly concerned about being able to find the cor-

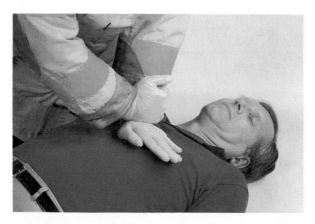

**Figure 7-9** Grasping the wrist of the hand positioned on the chest is an alternate hand position for giving chest compressions.

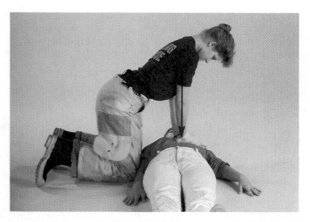

**Figure 7-10** With your hands in place, position yourself so that your shoulders are directly over your hands, arms straight and elbows locked.

rect position if the victim is obese, since fat does not accumulate over the sternum.

### Position of the Rescuer

Your body position is important when giving chest compressions. Compressing the chest straight down provides the best blood flow. The correct body position is also less tiring for you.

Kneel at the victim's chest with your hands in the correct position. Straighten your arms and lock your elbows so that your shoulders are directly over your hands (Fig. 7-10). When you press down in this position, you are pushing straight down onto the victim's sternum. Locking your elbows keeps your arms straight and prevents you from tiring quickly.

Compressing the chest requires little effort in this position. When you press down, the weight of your upper body creates the force needed to compress the chest. Push with the weight of your upper body, not with the muscles of your arms. Push straight down. Do not rock back and forth. Rocking results in less effective compressions and uses unnecessary energy. If your arms and shoulders tire quickly, you are not using the correct body position. After each compression, release the pressure

on the chest without losing contact with it and allow the chest to return to its normal position before you start the next compression (Fig. 7-11).

### Compression Technique

Each compression should push the sternum down from 1½ to 2 inches (3.8 to 5 cm). The downward and upward movement should be smooth, not jerky. Maintain a steady down-and-up rhythm, and do not pause between compressions. When you press down, the chambers of the heart empty. When you come up, release all pressure on the chest, which lets the chambers of the heart fill with blood between compressions.

Keep your hands in their correct position on the sternum. If your hands slip, find the notch as you did before and reposition your hands.

Give compressions at the rate of 80 to 100 per minute. As you do compressions, count aloud, "One and two and three and four and five and six and. . ." up to 15. Push down as you say the number and come up as you say "and." You should be able to do the 15 compressions in about 10 seconds. Even though you are compressing the chest at a rate of 80

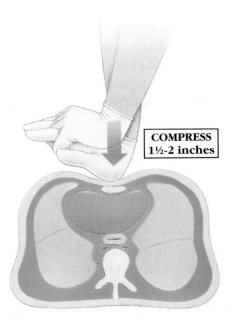

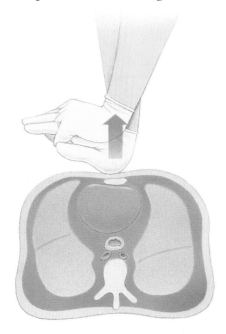

COMPRESS
1½-2 inches

**Figure 7-11** Push straight down with the weight of your body, then release, allowing the chest to return to the normal position.

to 100 times per minute, you will actually perform only 60 compressions in a minute. This is because you must take the time to do rescue breathing, giving 2 breaths between each group of 15 compressions.

## Compression/Breathing Cycles

When you give CPR, do cycles of 15 compressions and 2 breaths. You should be positioned midway between the chest and the head to move easily between compressions and breaths (Fig. 7-12). For each cycle, give 15 chest compressions, then open the airway with a head-tilt/chin-lift and give 2 slow breaths. This cycle should take about 15 seconds. When you are alone and using a resuscitation mask, the cycle may take longer. For each new cycle of compressions and breaths, use the correct hand position by first finding the notch at the lower end of the sternum.

After doing 4 cycles of continuous CPR, check to see if the victim's pulse has returned. These 4 cycles should take about 1 minute (Fig. 7-13). Tilt the victim's head to open the

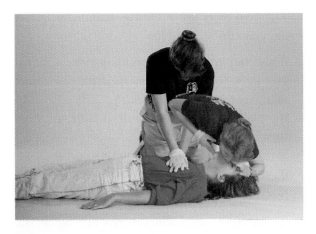

**Figure 7-12** Give 15 compressions, then give 2 breaths.

airway, and take time to check the carotid pulse. If there still is no pulse, continue CPR. Check the pulse again every few minutes. If you find a pulse, check for breathing. Give rescue breathing if necessary. If the victim is breathing, keep his or her airway open; continue to monitor breathing and pulse closely. (The Skill Sheets at the end of this chapter provide a step-by-step guide for CPR.)

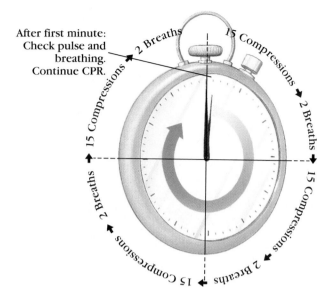

After first minute: Check pulse and breathing. Continue CPR.

2 Breaths · 15 Compressions · 2 Breaths · 15 Compressions · 2 Breaths · 15 Compressions · 2 Breaths · 15 Compressions

**Figure 7-13** Check the pulse at the end of the fourth cycle of 15 compressions and 2 breaths.

## When to Stop CPR

Once you begin CPR, try not to interrupt the blood flow you are creating artificially. However, you can stop CPR—

- ◆ If another trained person takes over CPR for you or if more advanced medical personnel take over care of the victim.
- ◆ If you are exhausted and unable to continue.
- ◆ If the scene suddenly becomes unsafe.
- ◆ If the person's heart starts beating adequately.

If the victim's heartbeat returns but he or she is still not breathing, continue giving rescue breathing. If the victim is breathing and has a heartbeat, keep the airway open and monitor breathing and pulse closely.

## ◆ CARDIAC EMERGENCIES IN INFANTS AND CHILDREN

A child's heart is usually healthy. Unlike adults, children do not often initially suffer a cardiac emergency. Instead, the child suffers a respiratory emergency and a cardiac emergency develops.

The most common cause of cardiac emergencies in children is injury from motor vehicle crashes. Other common causes for both infants and children include injuries from near-drowning, smoke inhalation, burns, poisoning, airway obstruction, firearms, and falls. Rarely, a cardiac emergency results from a medical condition or illness such as **croup** or **epiglottitis** (respiratory viral and bacterial infections that occur mainly in children and infants), or severe asthma.

Most cardiac emergencies in infants and children are preventable. Two ways to prevent them are to prevent injuries and make sure that infants and children receive proper medical care. A third way is to recognize the early signs of a respiratory emergency, which include—

- ◆ Agitation.
- ◆ Drowsiness.
- ◆ Change in skin color (to pale, blue, or gray).
- ◆ Increased difficulty breathing.
- ◆ Increased heart and breathing rates.

If you recognize that an infant or child is in respiratory distress or respiratory arrest, provide care immediately. If the infant or child is in cardiac arrest, start CPR immediately.

## ◆ CPR FOR INFANTS AND CHILDREN

The CPR technique for infants and children is similar to the technique for adults. As in rescue breathing, you need to modify the techniques to accommodate the smaller body size and faster breathing and heart rates. Figure 7-14 compares the adult, child, and infant CPR techniques.

## CPR for Children

To find out if a child needs CPR, begin with a primary survey. If you determine that there is no pulse, begin CPR.

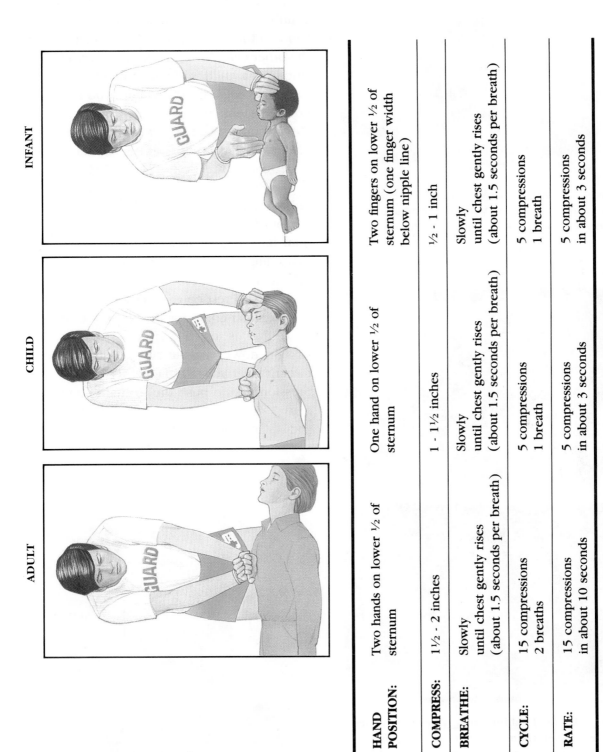

| | ADULT | CHILD | INFANT |
|---|---|---|---|
| **HAND POSITION:** | Two hands on lower ½ of sternum | One hand on lower ½ of sternum | Two fingers on lower ½ of sternum (one finger width below nipple line) |
| **COMPRESS:** | 1½ - 2 inches | 1 - 1½ inches | ½ - 1 inch |
| **BREATHE:** | Slowly until chest gently rises (about 1.5 seconds per breath) | Slowly until chest gently rises (about 1.5 seconds per breath) | Slowly until chest gently rises (about 1.5 seconds per breath) |
| **CYCLE:** | 15 compressions 2 breaths | 5 compressions 1 breath | 5 compressions 1 breath |
| **RATE:** | 15 compressions in about 10 seconds | 5 compressions in about 3 seconds | 5 compressions in about 3 seconds |

**Figure 7-14**   The technique for chest compressions differs for adults, children, and infants.

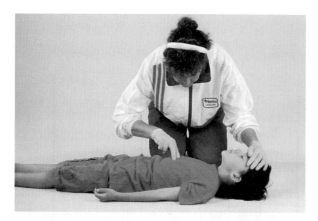

**Figure 7-15** While kneeling beside the child, maintain an open airway with one hand and find the correct hand position with the other.

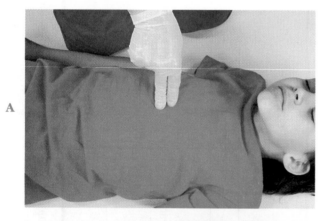

A

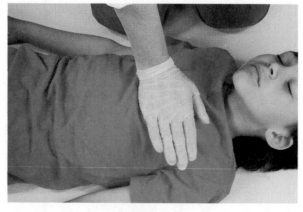

B

**Figure 7-16 A,** Find the notch where the lower rib meets the sternum with your middle finger. Place the index finger next to it, so that both fingers rest on the lower end of the breastbone. **B,** Place the heel of the same hand on the breastbone immediately above where you had your index finger.

To give compressions, kneel beside the child's chest with your knees against the child's side. Maintain an open airway with one hand and find the correct hand position with the other (Fig. 7-15). To locate your hand position on a child, slide your middle finger up the lower edge of the ribs until you locate the notch where the ribs meet the sternum (breastbone). Place the index finger next to it. The two fingers should be resting on the lower end of the sternum (Fig. 7-16, *A*).

Visually mark the place where you put your index finger. Lift your fingers off the sternum and put the heel of the same hand on the sternum immediately above where you had your index finger (Fig. 7-16, *B*). Keep your fingers off the child's chest. Only the heel of your hand should rest on the sternum.

When you compress the chest, use only the hand that is on the child's sternum. Push straight down, making sure your shoulder is directly over your hand (Fig. 7-17). Each compression should push the sternum down from 1 to 1½ inches (2.5 to 3.8 cm). The down-and-up movement should be smooth, not

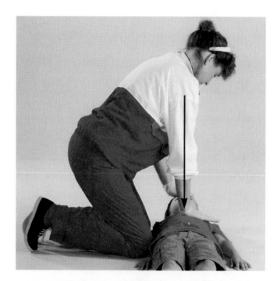

**Figure 7-17** When you compress the chest, use the heel of your hand. Push straight down, making sure your shoulder is directly over your hand.

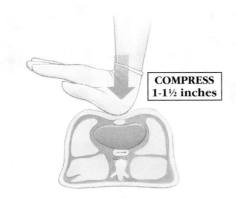
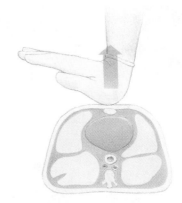

COMPRESS
1-1½ inches

**Figure 7-18** Push straight down with the weight of your body and then release, allowing the chest to return to its normal position.

jerky. Release the pressure on the chest completely, but do not lift your hand off the child's chest (Fig. 7-18).

When you give CPR to a child, do cycles of 5 compressions and 1 breath at a rate of about 100 compressions per minute. While giving compressions with one hand, keep your other hand on the child's forehead to help maintain an open airway. After giving 5 compressions, remove your compression hand from the chest, lift the chin, and give 1 slow breath. The breath should last about 1½ seconds. Always use a chin-lift with a head-tilt to ensure that the child's airway is open. After giving the breath, place your hand in the same position as before and continue compressions. You do not have to measure your hand position each time by sliding your fingers up the rib cage unless you lose your place.

Keep repeating the cycle of 5 compressions and 1 breath (Fig. 7-19). Each cycle of 5 compressions and 1 breath should take about 5 seconds. After you do about 1 minute of continuous CPR, recheck the child's pulse for about 5 seconds. If there is no pulse, continue CPR, starting with compressions. Repeat the pulse check every few minutes.

If you do find a pulse, then check for breathing. If the child is breathing, keep the airway open and monitor breathing and pulse closely. Check the pulse once every minute. If

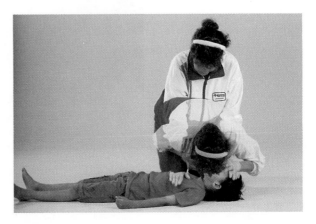

**Figure 7-19** Give 5 compressions and then 1 breath.

the child is not breathing, give rescue breathing and keep checking the pulse.

## CPR for Infants

To find out if an infant needs CPR, begin with a primary survey to check the ABCs. To check the pulse in an infant, locate the brachial pulse in the arm. If the infant has no pulse, begin CPR.

Position the infant faceup on a firm, flat surface. The infant's head must be on the same level as the heart or lower. Stand or kneel facing the infant from the side. Keep one hand on the infant's head to maintain an open airway. Use your other hand to give compressions.

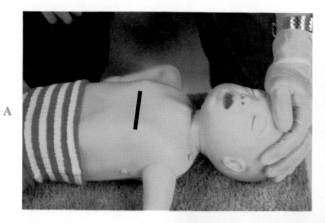
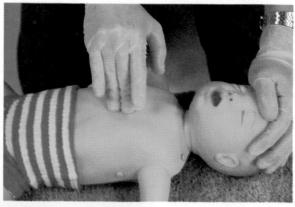
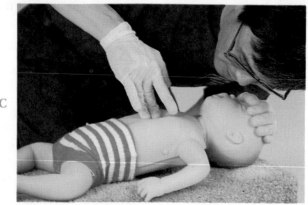

**Figure 7-20**  **A,** Imagine a line running across the chest between the infant's nipples. **B,** Place the middle and ring fingers next to your index finger on the breastbone. Raise the index finger. **C,** Use the pads of the remaining 2 fingers to compress the chest.

To find the correct place to give compressions, imagine a line running across the chest between the infant's nipples (Fig. 7-20, *A*). Place your index finger on the sternum (breastbone) just below this imaginary line. Then place 2 fingers next to your index finger on the sternum. Raise the index finger (Fig. 7-20, *B*). If you feel the notch at the end of the infant's sternum, move your fingers up a little bit.

Use the pads of fingers to compress the chest (Fig. 7-20, *C*). Compress the chest ½ to 1 inch, then let the sternum return to its normal position. When you compress, push straight down. The down-and-up movement of your compressions should be smooth, not jerky. Keep a steady rhythm. Do not pause between compressions. When you are coming up, release pressure on the infant's chest com-

pletely, but do not let your fingers lose contact with the chest (Fig. 7-21). Keep your fingers in the compression position. Use your other hand to keep the airway open using a head-tilt.

When you give CPR, do cycles of 5 compressions and 1 breath (Fig. 7-22). Compress at a rate of up to 120 compressions per minute, which is faster than the rate for an adult or a child. When you complete 5 compressions, give 1 slow breath, covering the infant's nose and mouth with your mouth. The breath should take about 1 to 1½ seconds. Keep repeating 5 compressions and 1 breath in about 5 seconds.

Recheck the pulse after about 1 minute of continuous CPR. Check the brachial pulse for about 5 seconds. If there is no pulse, continue CPR, starting with compressions. Repeat the

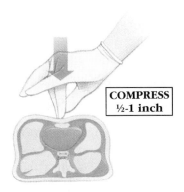
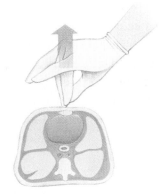

**Figure 7-21**  Push straight down with your fingers and then release the pressure on the chest completely.

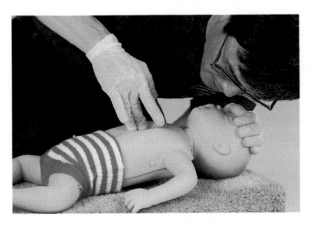

**Figure 7-22**  Give 5 compressions and then 1 breath.

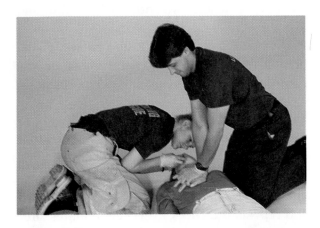

**Figure 7-23**  During two-rescuer CPR, the rescuers share the responsibility for performing rescue breathing and chest compressions.

pulse check every few minutes.

If you do find a pulse, then check breathing for about 5 seconds. If the infant is breathing, keep the airway open and monitor breathing and pulse closely. Check the pulse once every minute. Maintain normal body temperature. If the infant is not breathing, give rescue breathing.

### ◆ TWO-RESCUER CPR

When two professional rescuers are available, give two-rescuer CPR. You share the responsibility for performing rescue breathing and chest compressions (Fig. 7-23). You should be able to perform two-rescuer CPR in each of the following situations:

1. CPR is *not* being given, and two or more rescuers arrive on the scene at the same time and begin CPR together.
2. One rescuer is giving CPR, and a second rescuer is available to begin two-rescuer CPR.
3. Either rescuer tires and the rescuers change position.

### Two-Rescuer Techniques

In two-rescuer CPR for an adult, the victim is given breaths more often. Instead of the single-rescuer cycle of 15 compressions and two breaths, a two-rescuer CPR cycle involves 5 compressions and 1 breath (a ratio of 5 to 1). Compressions are stopped at the upstroke of the fifth compression, and the rescuer giving breaths immediately gives 1 slow breath for about 1½ seconds. The person giving compressions then continues.

Chest compressions are given at a rate of 80 to 100 per minute and at a depth of 1½ to 2 inches (3.8 to 5 cm), the same as in one-rescuer CPR for an adult or child. Rescuers use the same rhythm as for one-rescuer CPR: "One and two and three and four and five. . ." (breath) "One and two and three and four and five."

During two-rescuer CPR, the person giving breaths can check the effectiveness of the compressions by feeling for the carotid pulse while compressions are given (Fig. 7-24). Note that sometimes a carotid pulse may not be felt even though compressions are effective.

The rescuer giving breaths also does a pulse check after the first minute of compressions and repeats the check every few minutes after that to determine if circulation has returned. He or she says, "Pulse check," and compressions are stopped after the fifth compression. The pulse is checked for 5 seconds. If there

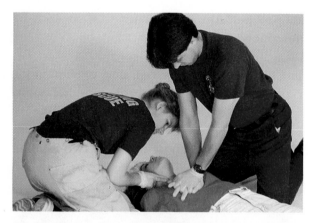

**Figure 7-24** The ventilator periodically checks the effectiveness of compressions by feeling for the carotid pulse while the compressor gives chest compressions.

is no pulse, continue CPR, starting with compressions.

## When Two Rescuers Arrive on the Scene at the Same Time

If CPR is not being performed when you arrive, one rescuer should do a primary survey and, if appropriate, begin CPR. The other rescuer should manage other responsibilities at the scene, such as scene safety, communications, and setting up equipment and supplies. Then the second rescuer can assist with CPR.

## Two Rescuers Beginning CPR Together

When both rescuers are available to begin CPR at the same time, the first rescuer does a primary survey. While the first rescuer is doing the primary survey, the second rescuer gets into position to give chest compressions and locates the correct hand position. He or she should begin chest compressions when the first rescuer says, "No pulse, begin CPR." Both rescuers continue CPR together.

## When CPR Is in Progress by One Rescuer

When a person is giving CPR and a second rescuer arrives, the second rescuer should first determine whether more advanced medical personnel have been summoned. If so, the second rescuer should either *replace* the first rescuer or *assist* him or her in giving two-rescuer CPR.

If the second rescuer is going to assist with two-rescuer CPR, he or she provides assistance after the first rescuer has completed a cycle of 15 compressions and 2 breaths.

The second rescuer gets into position at the victim's chest and finds the correct hand position. The first rescuer remains at the victim's head and checks the pulse. If there is still no pulse, the first rescuer signals to begin CPR.

The second rescuer at the chest begins chest compressions. Both rescuers continue giving two-rescuer CPR.

## Changing Positions

If a rescuer becomes tired, he or she can change positions with the other rescuer. When the rescuers change, the rescuer at the victim's head completes 1 breath and then moves immediately to the chest. The rescuer at the chest moves immediately to the head. Both rescuers move quickly into position without changing sides. The sequence for changing positions is the following:

1. The rescuer doing compressions says to change positions. He or she begins the cycle of compressions by saying, "Change and two and three and four and five."
2. Change positions. The rescuer at the head completes 1 breath at the end of the "change" cycle and moves to the chest. He or she locates the correct hand position and waits for the other rescuer to signal before beginning compressions. The other rescuer moves to the victim's head to give breaths. He or she checks for a pulse for 5 seconds. If there is no pulse, he or she says, "No pulse, continue CPR."
3. They continue two-rescuer CPR, each doing the task that the other person had been doing.

## ◆ PREVENTING CARDIOVASCULAR DISEASE

Although a heart attack seems to strike suddenly, the conditions that lead to it may develop over years. Many Americans' lifestyles may gradually be endangering their hearts, which can eventually result in cardiovascular disease. Potentially harmful behaviors frequently begin early in life. For example, many children develop tastes for "junk" foods that are high in cholesterol and have little or no nutritional value. Sometimes children are not encouraged to exercise.

Several studies have shown that coronary artery disease actually begins in the teenage years, when most smoking begins. Teenagers are more likely to begin smoking if their parents smoke. Smoking contributes to cardiovascular disease as well as to other diseases.

## Risk Factors for Heart Disease

Scientists have identified many factors, known as **risk factors,** that increase a person's chances of developing heart disease. Some risk factors for heart disease cannot be changed. For instance, men have a higher risk for heart disease than do women. A family history of heart disease also increases a family member's risk.

But people can control many risk factors for heart disease. Smoking, diets high in fats, high blood pressure, obesity, and lack of routine exercise are all linked to increased risk of heart disease. When one risk factor, such as high blood pressure, is combined with other risk factors, such as obesity or cigarette smoking, the risk of heart attack or stroke is greatly increased.

### Controlling Risk Factors

Controlling your risk factors involves adjusting your lifestyle to minimize the chance of future cardiovascular disease. The three major risk factors you can control are cigarette smoking, high blood pressure, and high blood cholesterol levels.

Cigarette smokers are more than twice as likely to have a heart attack as nonsmokers and two to four times as likely to have cardiac arrest. The earlier a person starts using tobacco, the greater the risk to his or her future health. Giving up smoking rapidly reduces the risk of heart disease. After a number of years,

## Healthy Heart IQ

The following statements represent a healthy lifestyle that can reduce your chances of heart disease. Check each statement that reflects your lifestyle.

I do not smoke and I avoid inhaling the smoke of others.

I eat a balanced diet that limits my intake of saturated fat and cholesterol.

I participate in continuous, vigorous physical activity for 20 to 30 minutes or more at least 3 times a week.

I have my blood pressure checked regularly.

I maintain an appropriate wieght.

If you did not check two or more of the statements, you should consider making changes in your lifestyle now. This chapter provides information on the subject of each statement.

the risk becomes the same as if the person had never smoked. If you do not smoke, do not start. If you do smoke, quit.

Uncontrolled high blood pressure can damage blood vessels in the heart, kidneys, and other organs. You can often control high blood pressure by losing excess weight and by changing your diet. When these are not enough, medications can be prescribed. It is important to have regular checkups to guard against high blood pressure and its harmful effects.

Diets high in saturated fats and cholesterol increase the risk of heart disease. These diets raise the level of cholesterol in the blood and increase the chances that cholesterol and other fatty materials will be deposited on blood vessel walls and cause atherosclerosis.

Some cholesterol in the body is essential. The amount of cholesterol in your blood is determined by how much your body produces and by the food you eat. Foods high in cholesterol include egg yolks, shrimp, lobster, and organ meats such as liver.

More important to an unhealthy blood cholesterol level is saturated fat. **Saturated fats** raise blood cholesterol level by interfering with the body's ability to remove cholesterol from the blood. Saturated fats are found in beef, lamb, veal, pork, ham, whole milk, and whole milk products.

Rather than eliminating saturated fats and cholesterol from your diet, limit your intake. This is easier than you may think; moderation is the key. Make changes whenever possible by substituting low-fat milk or skim milk for whole milk, margarine for butter, trimming visible fat from meats, and broiling or baking rather than frying. Read labels carefully. A "cholesterol-free" product may be high in saturated fat.

Two additional ways to help prevent heart disease are to control your weight and exercise regularly. Excess calories are stored as fat. In general, overweight people have a shorter life expectancy. Obese, middle-aged men have nearly three times the risk of a fatal heart attack as do normal-weight, middle-aged men.

Routine exercise has many benefits, including increased muscle tone and weight control. Exercise can also help you survive a heart attack because the increased circulation of blood through the heart develops additional channels for blood flow. If the primary channels that supply the heart are blocked in a heart attack, these additional channels can supply the heart tissue with oxygen-rich blood.

### Results of Managing Risk Factors

Managing the risk factors for cardiovascular disease really works. During the past 20 years, deaths from cardiovascular disease have decreased by 33 percent in the United States. As a result, as many as 250,000 lives may have been saved each year. Also, deaths from stroke have declined 50 percent.

Why did deaths from these causes decline? They probably declined as a result of improved detection and treatment, as well as lifestyle changes. People are becoming more aware of the risk factors for heart disease and are taking action to control them. If you do this, you can improve your chances of living a long and healthy life. If you suffer a cardiac arrest, your chances of survival are poor. Begin today to reduce your risk of cardiovascular disease. Completing the Healthy Heart IQ in this chapter will help you evaluate your risk for cardiovascular disease and other conditions that may cause sudden illness.

## ◆ SUMMARY

Being able to recognize signs and symptoms that may indicate a heart attack is important. If you think someone is suffering from a heart attack or if you are unsure, you should call for advanced medical care without delay. Begin care by having the victim stop what he or she is doing and rest in the most comfortable position possible.

When heartbeat and breathing stop, it is called *cardiac arrest*. A person who suffers a cardiac arrest is clinically dead, since no oxygen is reaching the cells of vital organs. Irreversible brain damage will occur from lack of oxygen. By starting CPR immediately, you can help keep the brain supplied with oxygen. By getting the victim advanced medical care, you can increase the cardiac arrest victim's chances for survival. If the victim does not have a pulse, start CPR. Always remember these simple guidelines for CPR:

- Use the correct hand position.
- Compress down and up smoothly.
- Combine compressions with ventilations.
- Repeat cycles of compressions and breaths.
- Recheck for the return of a pulse.
- If there is no pulse, continue CPR and recheck the pulse every few minutes.
- If the victim's pulse returns, stop CPR and check to see if the person has started to breathe.
- If the victim is still not breathing, begin rescue breathing.
- If two rescuers are available, begin two-rescuer CPR as soon as possible. If either of you tires, quickly change positions and continue.
- Once you start CPR, do not stop unnecessarily. Continue CPR until you are relieved by another trained person, you are exhausted, the victim's heart starts beating, or more advanced medical personnel arrive and take over.

## ◆ Review Questions ◆

Circle the letter of the best answer.

**1.** The purpose of cardiopulmonary resuscitation (CPR) is to—
a. Keep the brain supplied with oxygen until the heart can be restarted.
b. Prevent clinical death from occurring in a victim of cardiac arrest.
c. Restart heartbeat and breathing in a victim of cardiac arrest.
d. All of the above.

**2.** The most common cause of cardiac emergencies in children is—
a. Poisoning.
b. Near-drowning.
c. Motor vehicle injury.
d. Respiratory infection.

**3.** What should you do if a victim's breathing and heartbeat return while you are giving CPR?

  a. Have a bystander transport you and the victim to the nearest hospital.

  b. Continue rescue breathing while waiting for advanced medical personnel to arrive.

  c. Complete a secondary survey before calling more advanced medical personnel for assistance.

  d. Keep the airway open and monitor vitals signs.

**4.** During two-rescuer CPR, the person giving the breaths should—

  a. Count aloud to keep the person giving the compressions at the proper rate.

  b. Periodically check the effectiveness of the compressions by checking the carotid pulse during CPR.

  c. Call for a stop in the compressions after every minute to check for a return of pulse.

  d. All of the above.

**5.** The most prominent sign of a heart attack is—

  a. Difficulty breathing.

  b. Jaw and left arm pain.

  c. Nausea and sweating.

  d. Persistent chest pain.

**6.** In what position should you place a victim who may be experiencing a heart attack?

  a. The most comfortable position for the victim

  b. Sitting or semisitting

  c. Lying on the left side

  d. Lying on the back with legs elevated

**7.** High blood pressure can be controlled by—

  a. Losing excess weight.

  b. Changing dietary habits.

  c. Taking prescribed medication.

  d. All of the above.

**8.** Where should you place your hands to deliver effective chest compressions?

  a. Over the xiphoid process

  b. Over the lower half of the sternum

  c. On the middle of the sternum

  d. Just below the notch at the top of the sternum

**9.** Which is the primary sign of cardiac arrest?

  a. Absence of breathing

  b. Absence of blood pressure

  c. Absence of a carotid pulse

  d. Dilation of the pupils

**10.** To deliver chest compressions on a child, you would use the—

  a. Heel of one hand.

  b. Pads of two fingers.

  c. Heel of two hands.

  d. Pads of three fingers.

**Answers:** 1. a; 2. c; 3. d; 4. b; 5. d; 6. a; 7. d; 8. b; 9. c; 10. a.

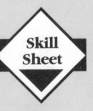
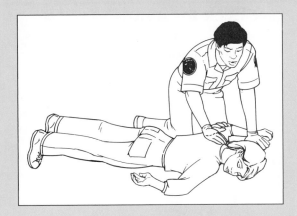

## ☐ Check for consciousness

- ◆ Tap or gently shake person.
- ◆ Shout, "Are you OK?"

**If person does not respond. . .**

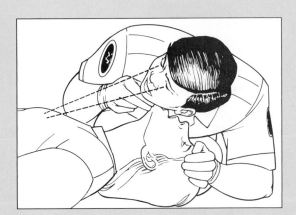

## ☐ Check for breathing

- ◆ Look, listen, and feel for about 5 seconds.

**If not breathing or you cannot tell . . .**

- ◆ Position victim on back. Roll person as a single unit while supporting the head and neck.
- ◆ Open the airway.
- ◆ Tilt head back and lift chin.
- ◆ Recheck breathing.
- ◆ Look, listen, and feel for about 5 seconds.

**If person is not breathing. . .**

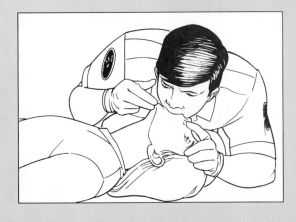

- ◆ Keep head tilted back.
- ◆ Pinch nose shut.
- ◆ Seal your lips tightly around person's mouth.
- ◆ Give 2 slow breaths, each lasting about 1½ seconds.
- ◆ Watch to see that the breaths go in.

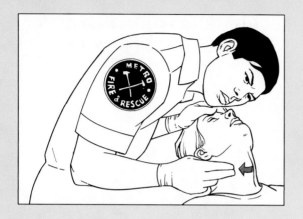

## ☐ Check for a pulse
- ◆ Locate Adam's apple.
- ◆ Slide fingers down into groove of neck on side closer to you.
- ◆ Feel for pulse for 5 to 10 seconds.

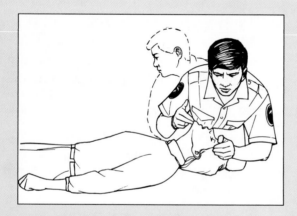

## ☐ Check for severe bleeding
- ◆ Look from head to toe for severe bleeding.

**If person does not have a pulse. . .**
- ◆ **Begin CPR.**

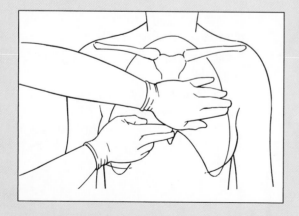

## ☐ Find hand position
- ◆ Locate notch at lower end of sternum.
- ◆ Place heel of other hand on sternum next to fingers.
- ◆ Remove hand from notch and put it on top of other hand.
- ◆ Keep fingers off chest.

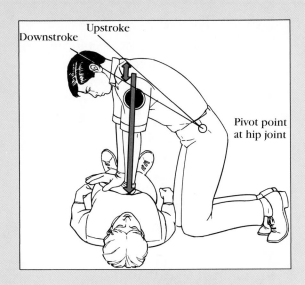

## ☐ Give 15 compressions

- ◆ Position shoulders over hands.
- ◆ Compress sternum 1½ to 2 inches.
- ◆ Do 15 compressions in about 10 seconds.
- ◆ Compress down and up smoothly, keeping hand contact with chest at all times.

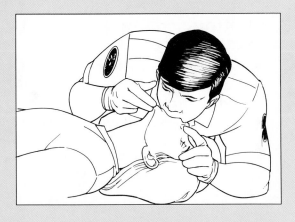

## ☐ Give 2 slow breaths

- ◆ Open airway with head-tilt/chin-lift.
- ◆ Pinch nose shut and seal your lips tightly around person's mouth.
- ◆ Give 2 slow breaths, each lasting about 1½ seconds.
- ◆ Watch chest to see that your breaths go in.

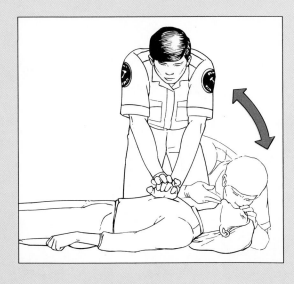

## ☐ Repeat compression/ breathing cycles

- ◆ Repeat cycles of 15 compressions and 2 breaths.

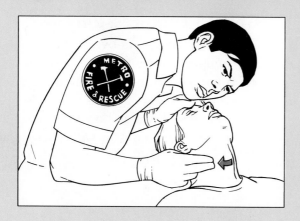

☐ **Recheck pulse**

- ◆ After about 1 minute, feel for pulse for about 5 seconds.

**If person has a pulse and is breathing. . .**

- ◆ Keep airway open.
- ◆ Monitor breathing.

**If person has a pulse but is still not breathing. . .**

- ◆ Do rescue breathing.

**If person does not have a pulse and is not breathing. . .**

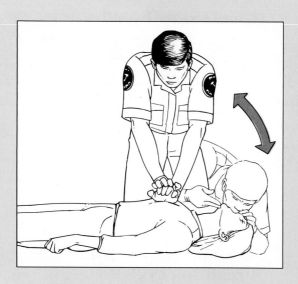

☐ **Continue compression/ breathing cycles**

- ◆ Locate correct hand position.
- ◆ Continue cycles of 15 compressions and 2 slow breaths.
- ◆ Recheck pulse and breathing every few minutes.

# CPR for a Child

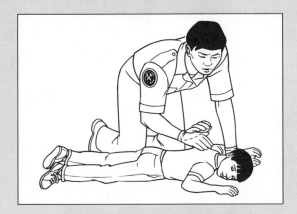

□ **Check for consciousness**

♦ Tap or gently shake child's shoulder.

**If child does not respond. . .**

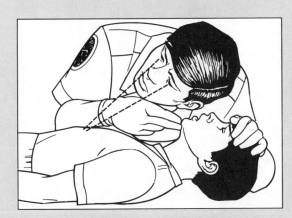

□ **Check for breathing**

♦ Look, listen, and feel for about 5 seconds.

**If not breathing or you cannot tell . . .**

♦ Position child on back. Roll child onto back while supporting the head and neck.
♦ Open the airway.
♦ Tilt head back and lift chin.
♦ Recheck breathing.
♦ Look, listen, and feel for about 5 seconds.

**If child is not breathing. . .**

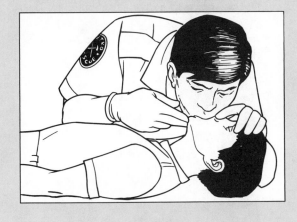

♦ Keep head tilted back.
♦ Seal your lips tightly around child's mouth.
♦ Give 2 slow breaths, each lasting about 1½ seconds.
♦ Watch to see that the breaths go in.

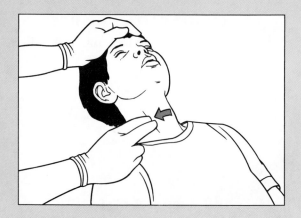

### ☐ Check for a pulse
- ◆ Locate carotid pulse.
- ◆ Slide fingers down into groove of neck on side closer to you.
- ◆ Feel for a pulse for 5 to 10 seconds.

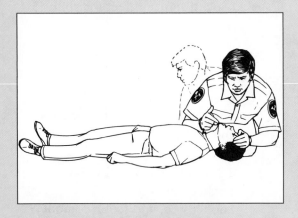

### ☐ Check for severe bleeding
- ◆ Look from head to toe for severe bleeding.

**If child does not have a pulse. . .**
- ◆ Begin CPR.

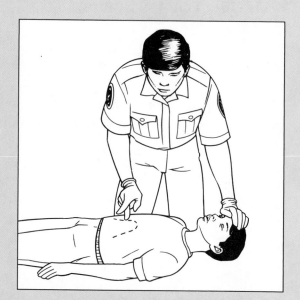

### ☐ Find hand position
- ◆ Maintain head-tilt with hand on forehead.
- ◆ Locate notch at lower end of sternum with other hand.

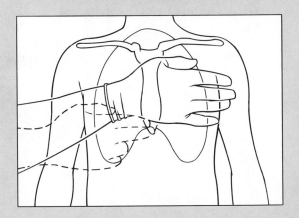

◆ Place heel of same hand on sternum immediately above where fingers were placed.

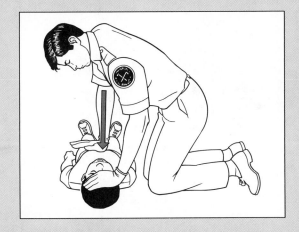

## ☐ Give 5 compressions

◆ Position shoulders over hands.
◆ Compress sternum 1 to 1½ inches.
◆ Do 5 compressions in about 3 seconds.
◆ Compress down and up smoothly, keeping hand contact with chest at all times.
◆ Maintain head-tilt with hand on forehead.

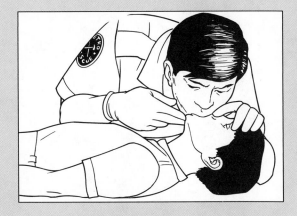

## ☐ Give 1 slow breath

◆ Open airway with head-tilt/chin-lift.
◆ Pinch nose shut and seal your lips tightly around child's mouth.
◆ Give 1 slow breath lasting about 1½ seconds.
◆ Watch chest to see that your breath goes in.

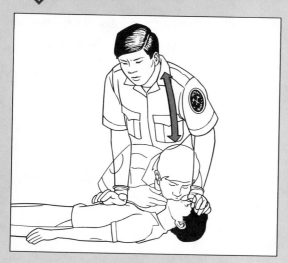

☐ **Repeat compression/ breathing cycles**

 ◆ Repeat cycles of 5 compressions and 1 breath.

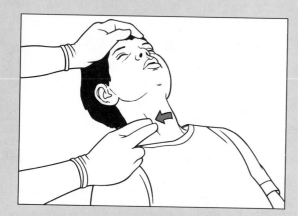

☐ **Recheck pulse**

 ◆ After about 1 minute, feel for pulse for about 5 seconds.

**If child has a pulse and is breathing. . .**

 ◆ Keep airway open.
 ◆ Monitor breathing.

**If child has a pulse but is still not breathing. . .**

 ◆ Do rescue breathing.

**If child does not have a pulse and is not breathing. . .**

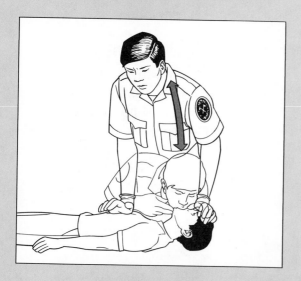

☐ **Continue compression/ breathing cycles**

 ◆ Locate correct hand position.
 ◆ Continue cycles of 5 compressions and 1 breath.
 ◆ Recheck pulse every few minutes.

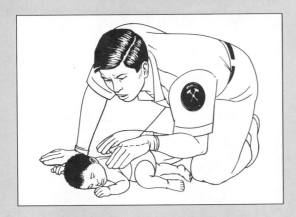

## ☐ Check for consciousness

♦ Tap or gently shake infant's shoulder.

**If infant does not respond. . .**

## ☐ Check for breathing

♦ Look, listen, and feel for about 5 seconds.

**If not breathing or you cannot tell. . .**

♦ Position infant on back. Roll infant onto back while supporting the head and neck.
♦ Open the airway.
♦ Tilt head back and lift chin.
♦ Recheck breathing.
♦ Look, listen, and feel for about 5 seconds.

**If infant is not breathing. . .**

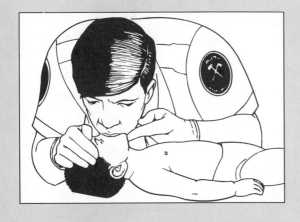

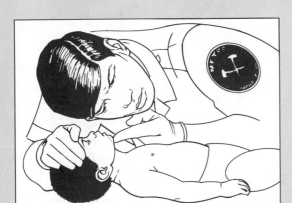

♦ Keep head tilted back.
♦ Seal your lips tightly around infant's mouth and nose.
♦ Give 2 slow breaths, each lasting about 1½ seconds.
♦ Watch to see that the breaths go in.

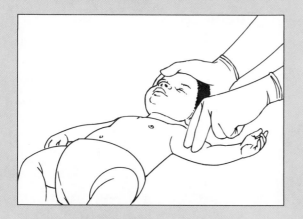

## ☐ Check for a pulse

- ◆ Locate brachial pulse.
- ◆ Place fingers on the inside of upper arm midway between elbow and shoulder.
- ◆ Feel for pulse for 5 to 10 seconds.

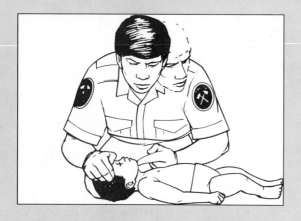

## ☐ Check for severe bleeding

- ◆ Look from head to toe for severe bleeding.

**If infant does not have a pulse. . .**
- ◆ **Begin CPR.**

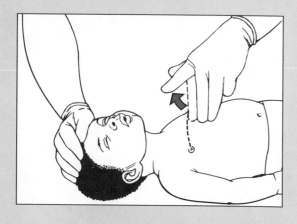

## ☐ Find hand position

- ◆ Maintain head-tilt with hand on fore-head.
- ◆ Place pads of fingers next to imaginary line running across chest connecting nipples.
- ◆ Raise your index finger.
- ◆ Adjust finger position if necessary.

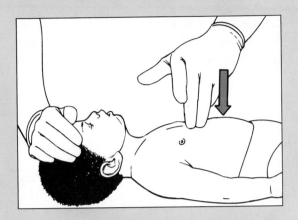

## Give 5 compressions

- Position hand over fingers.
- Compress sternum ½ to 1 inch.
- Do 5 compressions in about 3 seconds.
- Compress down and up smoothly, keeping finger in contact with chest at all times.
- Maintain head-tilt with hand on forehead.

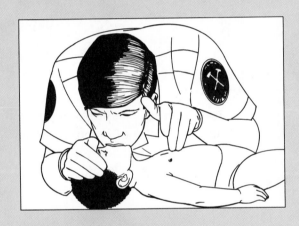

## Give 1 slow breath

- Maintain finger contact with chest.
- Seal your lips tightly around infant's mouth and nose.
- Give 1 slow breath lasting about 1½ seconds.
- Watch chest to see that your breath goes in.

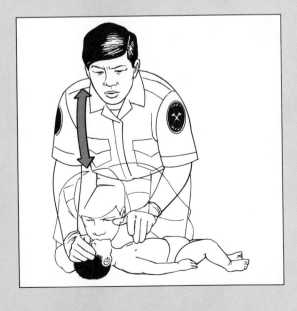

## Repeat compression/ breathing cycles

- Repeat cycles of 5 compressions and 1 breath.

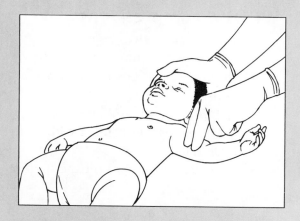

☐ **Recheck pulse**

- ♦ After about 1 minute, feel for brachial pulse for about 5 seconds.

**If infant has a pulse and is breathing. . .**

- ♦ Keep airway open.
- ♦ Monitor breathing.
- ♦ Wait for EMS personnel to arrive.

**If infant has a pulse but is still not breathing. . .**

- ♦ Do rescue breathing.

**If infant does not have a pulse and is not breathing. . .**

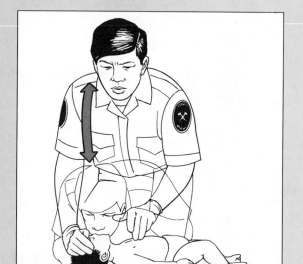

☐ **Continue compression/ breathing cycles**

- ♦ Locate correct compression position.
- ♦ Continue cycles of 5 compressions and 1 breath.
- ♦ Recheck pulse every few minutes.

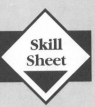
☐ **First rescuer—Complete primary survey**

- ◆ Check for consciousness.
- ◆ Position the person.

- ◆ Open airway and check for breathing.

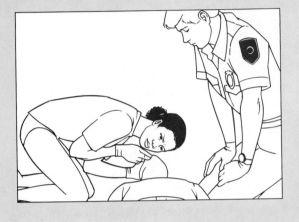

- ◆ Give 2 slow breaths.

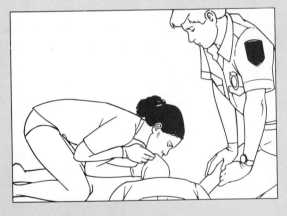

- ◆ Check for a pulse. Say, "No pulse."

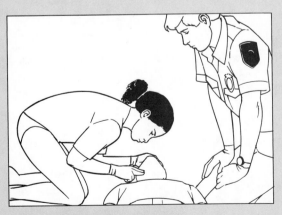

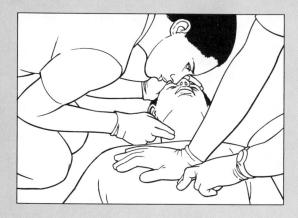

☐ **Second rescuer—Find hand position and give 5 compressions**

♦ Locate hand position while first rescuer checks pulse.

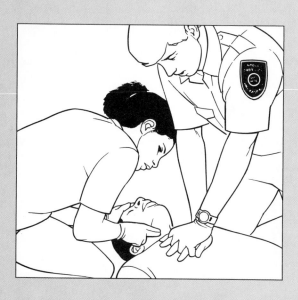

♦ Give 5 compressions in about 4 seconds, when first rescuer tells you to "Begin CPR."
♦ Count out loud, "One and, two and, three and, four and, five."
♦ Stop compressions and allow partner to ventilate.

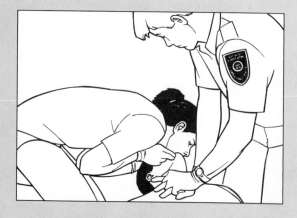

☐ **First rescuer—Give 1 slow breath**

♦ Give 1 slow breath lasting about 1½ seconds.

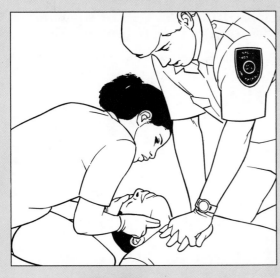

☐ **Both rescuers—Continue CPR**

♦ Repeat cycles of 5 compressions and 1 breath.

♦ Rescuer giving breaths—periodically check compression effectiveness by checking pulse while partner is giving compressions.

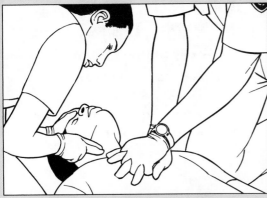

☐ **Recheck pulse and breathing**

♦ At end of first minute, check pulse for about 5 seconds.

**If person has a pulse. . .**

♦ Recheck breathing.

♦ If person is not breathing, do rescue breathing.

♦ Recheck pulse every minute.

**If person does not have a pulse. . .**

♦ Say, "No pulse, continue CPR."

♦ Continue CPR.

♦ Recheck pulse every few minutes.

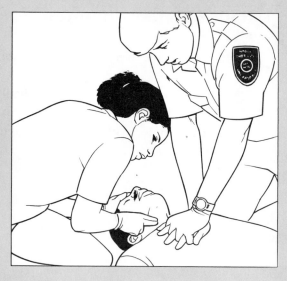

☐ **Compressor—Call for position change**

- ◆ Say, "Change and, two and, three and, four and, five."

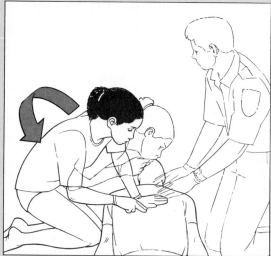

☐ **Both rescuers—Change positions**

**From ventilator to compressor—**

- ◆ Complete 1 slow breath at end of "change" cycle.
- ◆ Move quickly to person's chest.
- ◆ Find hand position. Wait for signal to begin compressions.

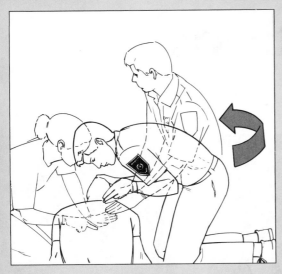

### From compressor to ventilator—

- ◆ Complete compression cycle.
- ◆ Move quickly to person's head and become ventilator.
- ◆ Feel for pulse for about 5 seconds.
- ◆ Say, "No pulse, continue CPR."

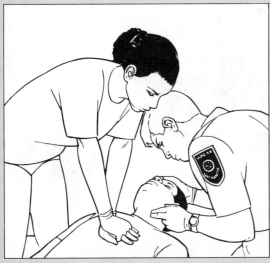

### ☐ Both rescuers—Continue CPR

- ◆ New compressor begins compressions.
- ◆ Both rescuers continue CPR with cycles of 5 compressions and 1 breath.
- ◆ New ventilator periodically checks for effectiveness of compressions and rechecks pulse and breathing every few minutes.

# Special Resuscitation Situations

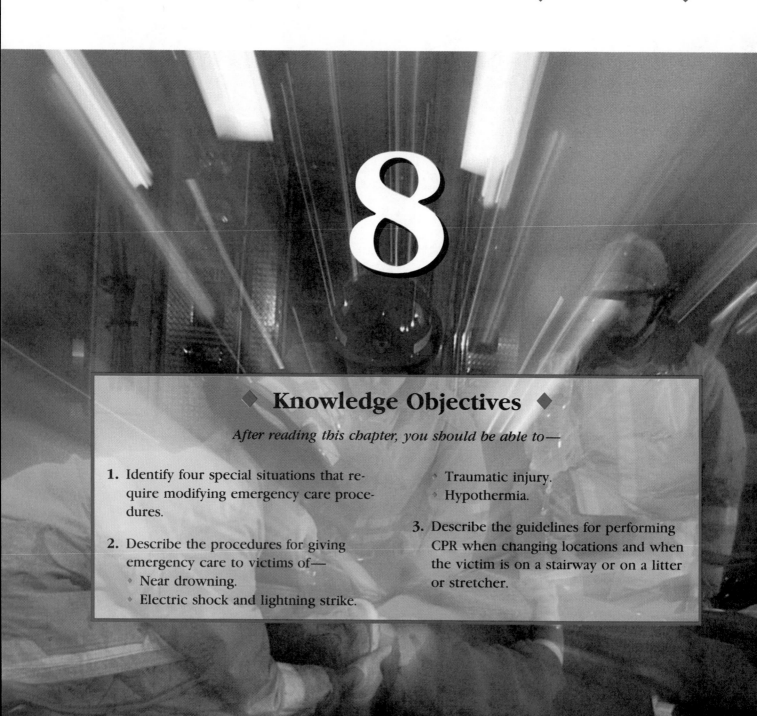

**8**

### ◆ Knowledge Objectives ◆

*After reading this chapter, you should be able to—*

1. Identify four special situations that require modifying emergency care procedures.

2. Describe the procedures for giving emergency care to victims of—
   - Near drowning.
   - Electric shock and lightning strike.

   - Traumatic injury.
   - Hypothermia.

3. Describe the guidelines for performing CPR when changing locations and when the victim is on a stairway or on a litter or stretcher.

◆ **Key Terms** ◆

Hypothermia: A life-threatening condition in which the entire body cools.

Near drowning: A situation in which a person who has been submerged in water survives.

Trauma: Physical injury caused by shock, pressure, or violence.

Trauma center: A medical facility specially equipped and staffed to give immediate emergency care to victims of traumatic injury.

◆ **Main Ideas** ◆

1. Certain situations, such as respiratory and/or cardiac arrest resulting from near drowning, electric shock and lightning strike, trauma, and hypothermia, require professional rescuers to change the emergency care procedures they normally use.

2. Professional rescuers may be required to perform CPR in unusual locations and situations that also require them to modify their usual emergency care techniques.

◆ **INTRODUCTION**

Some situations require the professional rescuer to change the emergency care procedures normally used. The most common special situations are—

◆ Near drowning.
◆ Electric shock and lightning strike.
◆ Traumatic injury.
◆ Hypothermia.

This chapter provides information about modifications the professional rescuer needs to make when providing rescue breathing and/or CPR in these situations. It also describes how to give CPR in difficult locations and situations.

◆ **NEAR DROWNING**

A person who has been submerged in water for more than 2 or 3 minutes will suffer from lack of oxygen and will need emergency care. The rescuer should get to the victim as soon as possible without risking personal safety. If possible, use something that floats, such as a life jacket, ring buoy, rescue tube, boat, raft, surfboard, and so on, to aid in the rescue (Fig. 8-1).

After reaching the victim, remove the victim from the water as quickly as possible. If you suspect the victim may have a head or spine injury, you must support the victim's neck and keep it aligned with the body. If it is necessary to turn the victim on his or her back, the victim's head, neck, chest, and the rest of the body must be aligned, supported, and turned as a unit (Fig. 8-2). The victim should be floated on his or her back onto a firm support such as a backboard or a surfboard before being moved from the water (Fig. 8-3).

Once the victim is out of the water, open the airway and check for breathing. Begin ventilation if the victim is not breathing. If you are unable to get air into the victim, the airway is probably obstructed. In this case, give abdominal thrusts. Before giving thrusts turn the victim's head to one side, unless you suspect head or spine injury. Doing this will allow water or vomit to drain from the mouth. Once you have been able to get your air in, check circulation.

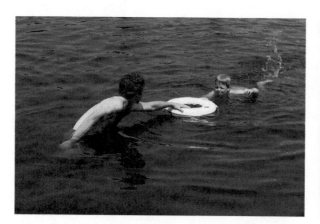 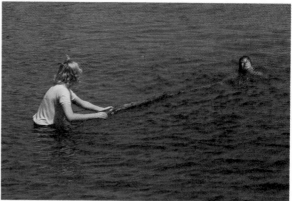

**Figure 8-1**   If you can enter the water without endangering yourself, wade out toward the victim and extend an object for the victim to grasp.

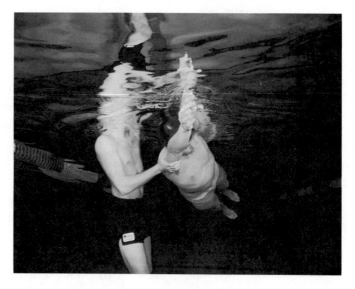

**Figure 8-2**   If you have to turn the victim onto the back, align all parts of the body and turn the body as a unit.

The pulse may be difficult to detect in a **near-drowning** victim and may have to be checked a little longer. If you cannot feel a pulse, start CPR. Performing chest compressions in the water is not practical. The body needs to be on a hard, firm, horizontal surface for compressions to be effective.

Basic life support should be continued until more advanced medical help is available. Every near-drowning victim, regardless of how rapid the recovery, should be transported to a medical facility immediately for follow-up care.

You should attempt to resuscitate the victim even if he or she has been submerged for a prolonged period. People have been successfully resuscitated even after being submerged for longer than 30 minutes. Continue CPR until advanced care can be started.

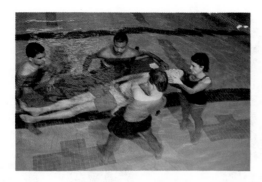

**Figure 8-3** To float the victim onto a backboard, submerge the backboard and move it under the victim.

## ◆ ELECTRIC SHOCK AND LIGHTNING STRIKE

### Electric Shock

Electric shock causes between 500 and 1,000 deaths each year in the United States; 5,000 additional victims have to receive emergency treatment. Electricity can seriously burn victims. Electric shock can also paralyze the breathing muscles, causing cardiac arrest.

The length of contact with the source of electricity, the strength of the current, and the environmental conditions all affect the severity of an electric shock. Immediately following severe electric shock, the victim may not be breathing and may not have a pulse. Remember, however, that it is critically important that attempts to reach and resuscitate the victim do not put you or anyone else in danger. No one should approach the victim until the source of the electricity is turned off. If the shock has been caused by downed electric power lines, contact the power company.

Once you reach the victim, immediately check the airway, breathing, and circulation. Start rescue breathing or CPR at once if the victim is not breathing or has no pulse.

A person who receives a shock while working in a high or hard-to-reach location, such as a utility pole, and is no longer breathing, should be given rescue breathing immediately, provided he or she is not in contact with the electrical source. The victim should be lowered to the ground at once, and CPR should be started immediately as soon as the victim is faceup on a hard, firm surface.

### Lightning Strike

Lightning kills from 50 to 300 people a year in the United States and seriously injures about twice that many. It acts as a direct current that interrupts the heart's rhythm. Victims most likely to die of lightning injury are those who suffer immediate cardiac arrest. Those whose heart does not stop have an excellent chance of recovery.

Efforts to resuscitate lightning victims may be successful even when some time has passed before the attempts are initiated. Lightning can also cause fractures, including spinal fracture, and severe burns.

## ◆ TRAUMATIC INJURY

Survival rates from cardiac arrest as a result of trauma are extremely poor. For this reason the victim must be transported to a **trauma center** as soon as possible for specialized treatment. Airway management should be rapidly initiated. Intubation of the trachea is a priority for those trained in such techniques. Chest compressions are of unknown value for such victims.

Use care not to further injure a trauma victim at the scene of an accident. You should suspect head or spine injury in a trauma victim, especially one whose injuries were the result of a vehicle accident, a fall from a height, or a diving or skiing accident.

While attempting to open the airway, be sure that the victim's head and neck are stabilized (Fig. 8-4).

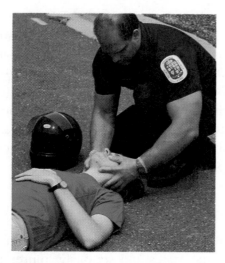

**Figure 8-4** Support the victim's head in line with the body.

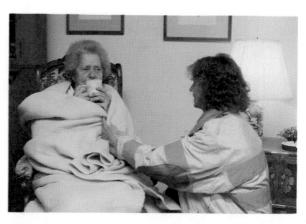

**Figure 8-5** Rewarm the body of a hypothermia victim gradually.

## ◆ HYPOTHERMIA

In **hypothermia** the entire body cools and body temperature falls below 95 degrees Fahrenheit (35 degrees C). Severe hypothermia occurs when the body temperature drops below 86 degrees Fahrenheit (30 degrees C). The victim will die if not given care. As the body temperature cools, blood flow to the brain decreases, the body's oxygen requirements become less, and blood pressure falls. The heart begins to beat erratically, and the victim can go into cardiac arrest. Pulse and breathing can become hard to detect, the body may feel stiff as the muscles become rigid, and the victim may appear to be dead.

Rescue breathing should be started immediately if the victim is not breathing. Before starting CPR, check the victim's pulse for up to 45 seconds. If you cannot detect a pulse, begin CPR. The victim should be transported at once to a medical facility for follow-up care and should continue to receive CPR on the way. Prevent further heat loss by removing any wet clothing and protecting the victim from wind or cold. Warm the body gradually by wrapping the victim in blankets or dry clothing (Fig. 8-5). You can apply warm packs

or hot water bottles to the neck, armpits, and groin. Rapid rewarming and rough handling can cause dangerous heart rhythms, so handle the victim gently and rewarm gradually.

The air temperature does not have to be below freezing for people to develop hypothermia (Fig. 8-6). Elderly people in poorly heated homes, particularly people who lack proper nutrition and exercise, can develop hypothermia at higher temperatures. The homeless and ill are also at risk. Certain substances, such as alcohol and barbiturates, can also interfere with the body's normal response to cold, causing hypothermia to occur more easily. Medical conditions, such as infection, insulin reaction, stroke, and brain tumor, also make a person more susceptible. Anyone remaining in cold water or wet clothing for a prolonged time may also easily develop hypothermia.

## ◆ CPR IN DIFFICULT LOCATIONS AND SITUATIONS

Professional rescuers often find themselves working under unique or unusual circumstances. It is common to perform CPR in bath-

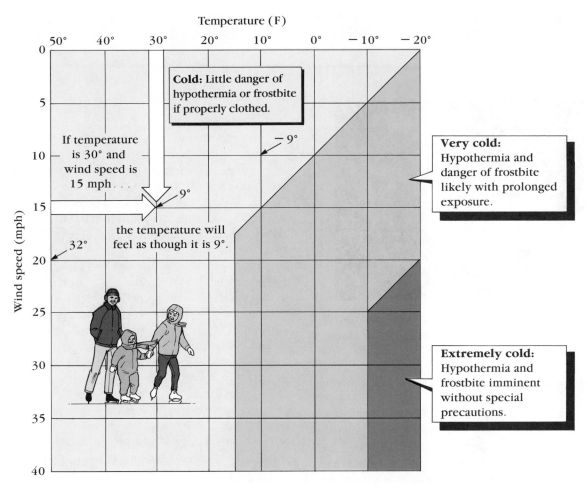

**Temperature (F)**

Cold: Little danger of hypothermia or frostbite if properly clothed.

If temperature is 30° and wind speed is 15 mph . . .

— 9°

Very cold: Hypothermia and danger of frostbite likely with prolonged exposure.

9°

the temperature will feel as though it is 9°.

32°

Extremely cold: Hypothermia and frostbite imminent without special precautions.

Wind speed (mph)

**Figure 8-6**  Low temperature and high wind increase the chance for hypothermia to occur.

rooms, in elevators, on subway platforms, and in moving vehicles. Use the following guidelines:

◆ Only move a victim from a cramped or busy location if it is unsafe or impractical to perform CPR.

◆ In some instances, a victim has to be transported up or down a flight of stairs. It is best to perform CPR at the head or foot of the stairs. Then, using a predetermined signal, interrupt CPR, move quickly to the next level, and resume CPR. Interruptions should not last longer than 30 seconds and should be avoided if possible.

◆ CPR should not be interrupted while a victim is being transferred to an ambulance or into the emergency department. With a low-wheeled litter, you can stand alongside

and perform compressions as you walk beside the litter. With a high litter or bed, you may have to kneel beside the victim on the bed or litter, or stand on a stool next to the bed or litter rails to get sufficient height to compress the chest adequately.

## ◆ SUMMARY

Certain situations may require the professional rescuer to change or modify emergency care procedures. These situations include near drowning, electric shock and lightning strike, traumatic injury, and hypothermia. Professional rescuers should also be prepared to cope with occasions when a victim is in a cramped or busy location, on a stairway, or on a bed or litter.

# Striking Distance

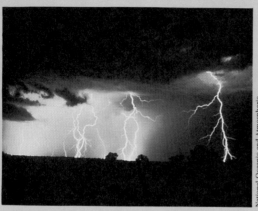

National Oceanic and Atmospheric Administration (NOAA)

In medieval times, people believed that ringing church bells would dissipate lightning during thunderstorms. It was an unfortunate superstition for the bell ringers. Over 33 years, lightning struck 386 church steeples and 103 bell ringers died.[1]

Church bell ringers have dropped off the list of people most likely to be struck during a thunderstorm, but lightning strikes remain extremely dangerous. Lightning causes more deaths annually in the United States than any other weather hazard, including blizzards, hurricanes, floods, tornadoes, earthquakes, and volcanic eruptions. The National Weather Service estimates that lightning kills nearly 100 people annually and injures about 300 others. Lightning occurs when particles of water, ice, and air moving inside storm clouds lose electrons. Eventually, the cloud becomes divided into layers of positive and negative particles. Most electrical currents run between the layers inside the cloud. However, occasionally, the negative charge flashes toward the ground, which has a positive charge. An electrical current snakes back and forth between the ground and the cloud many times in the seconds that we see a flash crackle down from the sky. Anything tall—a tower, a tree, or a person—becomes a path for the electrical current.

Traveling at speeds up to 300 miles per second, a lightning strike can hurl a person through the air, burn his or her clothes off, and sometimes cause the heart to stop beating. The most severe lightning strikes carry up to 50 million volts of electricity, enough to keep 13,000 homes running. Lightning can "flash" over a person's body, or, in its more dangerous path, it can travel through blood vessels and nerves to reach the ground.

Besides burns, lightning can also cause neurologic damage, fractures, and loss of hearing or eyesight. The victim sometimes acts confused and amnesiac and may describe the episode as getting hit on the head or hearing an explosion.

Use common sense around thunderstorms. If you see a storm approaching in the distance, do not wait until you are drenched to seek shelter. If a thunderstorm threatens, the National Weather Service advises you to—

- Go inside a large building or home.
- Get inside a car and roll up the windows.
- Stop swimming or boating as soon as you see or hear a storm. Water conducts electricity.
- Stay away from the telephone, except in an emergency.
- Stay away from telephone poles and tall trees if you are caught outside.
- Stay off hilltops; try to crouch down in a ravine or valley.
- Stay away from farm equipment and small metal vehicles such as motorcycles, bicycles, and golf carts.
- Avoid wire fences, clotheslines, metal pipes and rails, and other conductors.
- Stay several yards apart if you are in a group.

## REFERENCES

1. Kessler E: *The thunderstorm in human affairs,* Norman, Oklahoma, 1983, University of Oklahoma.
2. Randall T: 50 million volts may crash through a lightning victim, *The Chicago Tribune,* Section 2 D, August 13, 1989.

# ◆ Review Questions ◆

**1.** Chest compressions for a near-drowning victim—
a. Should be given while the victim is in the water.
b. Are not effective unless the victim is on a hard, firm surface.
c. Should be given along with rescue breathing.
d. b and c.

**2.** You are summoned to a scene where a lineman has received a severe electric shock and is still on the pole. Your first action is—
a. To bring him down from the pole immediately.
b. To give him rescue breathing while he is still on the pole.
c. To check the victim's pulse.
d. To make sure the victim is not in contact with the power source and it is safe for you to help.

**3.** When a victim of an automobile accident is still in the car, you remove the victim—
a. If the victim is conscious.
b. If you must to provide care.
c. If the victim asks to be moved.
d. If you suspect head or spine injury.

**4.** For a victim of hypothermia, you should—
a. Remove any wet clothing.
b. Warm the victim gradually and handle gently.
c. Check for a pulse for as long as 45 seconds.
d. All of the above.

**5.** When transporting a person without a pulse down a stairway—
a. Give CPR, then move the victim and resume CPR within 30 seconds.
b. Give rescue breathing at once but no compressions until the victim is off the stairs.
c. Get the victim off the stairs before giving CPR.
d. Give CPR on the stairs until more advanced medical help arrives.

**Answers:** 1. d; 2. d; 3. b; 4. d; 5. a.

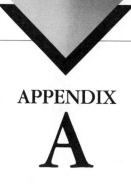

# A

# Automated External Defibrillation (AED)

## ◆ INTRODUCTION

Each year, over 500,000 Americans experience a heart attack. More than 300,000 of these attacks result in sudden death—cardiac arrest. Most of these arrests occur away from a hospital, where the care needed to immediately correct the cardiac arrest condition is not readily available. CPR, started promptly, can help. However, CPR by itself is insufficient to correct the underlying heart problem. What is needed to correct the problem, in more than two thirds of all cardiac arrests, is an electric shock. And the sooner the shock is administered, the greater the likelihood of the victim's survival.

In the prehospital setting, this shock, known as **defibrillation,** has generally been administered only by paramedics. However, paramedics are rarely the first to arrive on the emergency scene. Often, basic EMTs and first responders, such as fire fighters and law enforcement personnel, arrive first. But without the capability to defibrillate, they are limited to performing CPR while awaiting the arrival

of more advanced personnel. This delay in defibrillation is believed to be a major contributing factor to the low survival rate associated with out-of-hospital cardiac arrest.

As a result, the medical community is focusing efforts on providing earlier defibrillation to cardiac arrest victims. To make this possible, both the defibrillator and the skills needed to operate one properly have been simplified. This has resulted in more individuals being able to defibrillate cardiac arrest victims and more victims of cardiac arrest being saved. This appendix has been developed to help orient professional rescuers to the need for early defibrillation programs and the basic principles of how automated defibrillation works.

## ◆ THE HEART'S ELECTRICAL SYSTEM

To better understand both the limitations of CPR and how defibrillation works, it is helpful to understand how the heart's electrical sys-

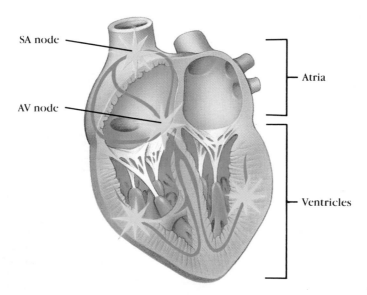

**Figure AA-1** The Conduction System of the Heart

tem functions. This electrical system determines the pumping action of the heart. Under normal conditions, specialized cells of the heart initiate and carry on electrical activity. These cells make up what is commonly called *the conduction system*. Think of the conduction system as the pathway or road that electrical impulses must travel. This pathway originates in the upper chambers of the heart, known as the *atria*. It ends in the lower chambers of the heart, known as the *ventricles* (Fig. AA-1).

The exact point of origin of the electric impulse is the sinoatrial node, commonly called the *SA node*. Approximately every second of an adult's life, a new electrical impulse is generated from the SA node. This impulse travels down the pathway of cells to a point midway between the atria and ventricles. This point is the atrioventricular node, commonly called the *AV node*.

Below the AV node, the pathway divides like a fork in a road into two branches. The electrical impulse travels by way of these right and left branches to its final destination, the right and left ventricles. Through a vast network of microscopic fibers, called *Purkinje fi-*

*bers*, the impulse reaches the muscular walls of the ventricles where it causes the ventricles to contract. The strong contraction of the ventricles forces blood out of the heart to circulate through the body, resulting in a pulse. The pauses between the pulse beats you feel are the periods between contractions.

Through the timing of these electrical impulses, the chambers of the heart are able to contract and relax. When they contract, blood is forced out of the heart. When they relax, blood refills the chambers.

The electrical activity of the heart can be evaluated by a cardiac monitor. The cardiac monitor has electrodes that usually are attached to the chest. The electrodes pick up the electrical impulse and transmit it to the monitor. The movement of the electrical impulse down the pathway appears as a tracing on the monitor. This tracing is referred to as an **electrocardiogram (ECG).** A regular rhythm that occurs within a normal rate, 60 to 100 beats per minute (bpm), and without unusual variations, is called a **normal sinus rhythm.** This rhythm appears on an ECG as a series of regularly spaced and sized peaks and valleys (Fig. AA-2, *A*).

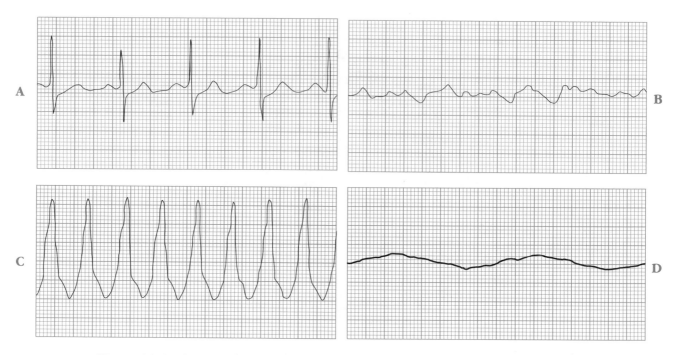

**Figure AA-2** **A,** Normal sinus rhythm. **B,** Ventricular fibrillation (V-fib). **C,** Ventricular tachycardia (V-tach). **D,** Asystole.

## ◆ WHEN THE HEART FAILS

Any damage to the heart, caused either by disease or injury, can disrupt the conduction system. This can result in an abnormal heart rhythm that can stop circulation. The most common abnormal rhythm, present initially in cardiac arrest victims, is **ventricular fibrillation (V-fib).** This is a state of totally disorganized electrical activity in the heart (Fig. AA-2, *B*). It results in the fibrillation, or quivering, of the ventricles. This fibrillation is not adequate for the ventricles to pump blood. Consequently, there is no pulse.

Another abnormal rhythm is **ventricular tachycardia,** commonly called **V-tach.** The term *tachycardia* means fast heart. V-tach, therefore, refers to a very rapid contraction of the ventricles. Though there is electrical activity resulting in a regular rhythm, the rate is often so fast that the heart is unable to pump blood properly (Fig. AA-2, *C*). As with V-fib, when blood flow is severely impaired, there will not be a pulse.

In many cases, these two abnormal rhythms can be corrected by early defibrillation. During defibrillation, an electrical shock is delivered to the heart. This shock is not intended to start a dead heart, one without any electrical activity. Instead, it is intended to disrupt abnormal electrical activity, such as that of V-fib and V-tach, long enough to allow the heart to spontaneously develop an effective rhythm on its own.

If not interrupted, these rhythms will deteriorate to the point where all electrical activity will cease, a condition known as **asystole** (Fig. AA-2, *D*). Asystole is not corrected by defibrillation and indicates a dead heart, which is extremely unlikely to be resuscitated.

CPR, begun immediately and continued until defibrillation is available, will help prolong V-fib so that it can be corrected by defibrillation. In addition, CPR performed during this period appears to contribute to preserving brain function. However, CPR cannot maintain V-fib indefinitely and cannot convert V-fib to a normal sinus rhythm. The major factor determining survival for a person in V-fib is the time until defibrillation. The longer the wait, the poorer the outcome. For this reason, programs teaching and promoting early defibrillation to more emergency care providers are encouraged.

## ◆ AUTOMATED EXTERNAL DEFIBRILLATORS: IMPROVING SURVIVAL OF CARDIAC ARREST

The use of the traditional manual defibrillator requires specialized training that includes learning how to recognize abnormal rhythms on a monitor and how to deliver a shock with hand-held paddles. The process not only demands extensive training, but the manual defibrillators are expensive. It is, therefore, impractical to train first responders in their use.

Instead, the answer to the problem of how to get timely, lifesaving defibrillation to cardiac arrest victims sooner lies with **automated external defibrillators (AEDs)** (Fig. AA-3). As the name implies, the AED is an automatic device. Some devices are considered "fully automatic"; others are "semiautomatic." When properly applied, both devices are capable of automatically recognizing a heart rhythm that requires a shock. A fully automatic device then charges itself and delivers a

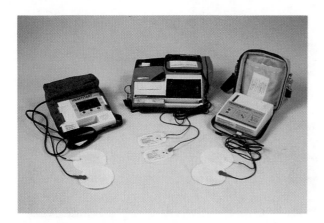

**Figure AA-3** Automated External Defibrillators

shock to the victim. The semiautomatic device advises the rescuer to push a button to deliver the shock.

Not only are both of these devices simple to operate, they are also extremely reliable. Studies have shown that AEDs analyze the victim's heart rhythm several times before identifying it as one for which a shock is indicated. In addition, the devices are not misled by movement, such as that of a victim having a seizure.

## Using an Automated External Defibrillator

In a situation involving cardiac arrest, an AED should be put to use as soon as it is available. Other skills, such as CPR already in progress, must be stopped once the AED is applied. All AEDs, regardless of whether they are fully automatic or semiautomatic, can be operated by following four simple steps:

1. Check for the absence of a pulse to confirm cardiac arrest.
2. Turn on the AED.
3. Attach the device to the victim.
4. Deliver a shock, if indicated.

Whether you are the first person to arrive on the scene or arrive after CPR has been started, you should check the victim's pulse to determine that the victim is actually in cardiac arrest before attaching the AED (Fig. AA-4). The absence of a pulse confirms cardiac arrest. At this point, you should turn on the AED (Fig. AA-5). Once the device is turned on, a microcassette tape deck begins recording the voices and sounds from the surrounding area. At this point, you briefly give a verbal report for the recording. It should include—

* Your identity and location.
* Assessment findings.
* Any significant events that have occurred (for example, drowning incident, trauma).

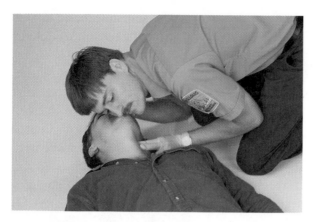

**Figure AA-4** Before attaching the AED, you should always check the victim's pulse to determine that the victim is in cardiac arrest.

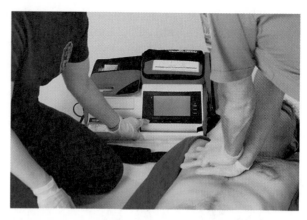

**Figure AA-5** After you have confirmed that the victim is in cardiac arrest, turn on the AED.

Next, prepare to attach the necessary equipment to the victim. Attaching the device to the victim requires that you apply two adhesive pads to the victim's chest. To do this, the victim's chest must be bare and wiped dry. Remove the pads from their packaging. Connect the two cables from the AED to the pads (Fig. AA-6, *A*). The cables are color-coded (red or white).

Peel away the protective plastic backing from the pads (Fig. AA-6, *B*). Place the pads, adhesive-side down, on the victim's chest. Place one pad connected to the white cable on the upper right side of the victim's chest,

between the nipple and the collarbone. Place the other pad connected to the red cable on the lower left side of the victim's chest, below the nipple (Fig. AA-7). If you are confused about which pad goes where, remember the phrase "white goes upper right." This means that the pad attached to the white cable is applied to the upper right side of the victim's chest.

If the pads are not securely attached to the chest or if the cables are not fastened properly, you will receive an "error" or "no contact" message from the AED. This may appear in print on the small screen on the front of the

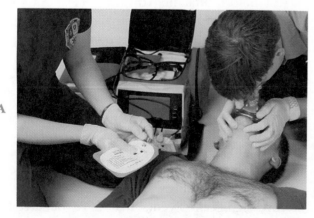
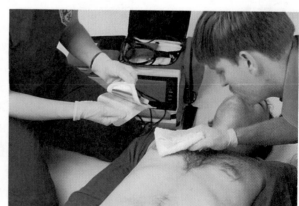

**Figure AA-6** **A,** Connect the two cables from the AED to the pads. **B,** Peel away the protective backing from the pads.

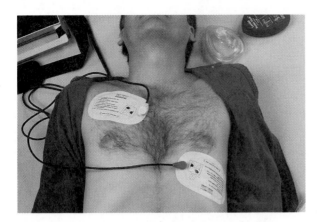

**Figure AA-7** Place the pad connected to the white cable on the right side of the chest between the nipple and collarbone. Place the pad connected to the red cable on the left side of the chest below the nipple.

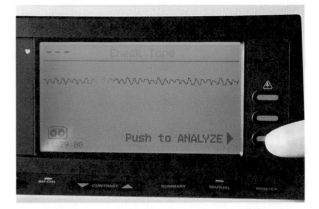

**Figure AA-8** When using a semiautomatic device, press the button marked "analyze."

machine. If this happens, check to see that the pads and cables are attached properly. In all cases, you should follow the manufacturer's instructions, since AEDs differ in the type of cables and adhesive pads used.

At this point, the device is ready to analyze the heart rhythm. If you are using a semiautomatic device, you will need to press the button marked "analyze" to have the machine examine the heart rhythm (Fig. AA-8). If the AED identifies a rhythm that should be defibrillated, it will prompt you with either an on-screen message or by voice synthesizer. This prompt often states, "shock advised," indicating that

you need to press a button to defibrillate the victim (Fig. AA-9). The fully automatic AED will analyze the heart rhythm, charge to the appropriate energy level, advise you that a shock is needed, and deliver a shock of the correct intensity automatically.

You will also be instructed by a voice message within the AED to "stand clear" before administering a shock. This is an important measure that you and others present must follow. Any time an AED is analyzing the rhythm, charging to a specific energy level, or administering a shock, you and others must *not* be in contact with the victim (Fig. AA-10). It is the

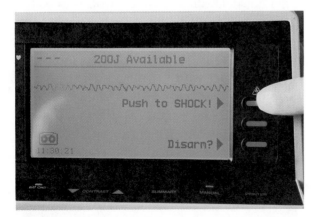

**Figure AA-9** The AED will prompt you when to administer the shock.

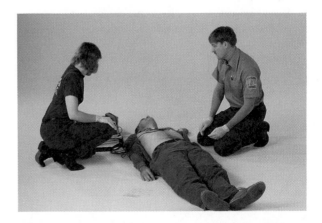

**Figure AA-10** Everyone must "stand clear" when the AED is analyzing the rhythm, charging the energy level, and administering a shock.

responsibility of the operator to move rescuers away from contact with the victim before analyzing and before depressing the shock button. This can be done by shouting "stand clear."

---

**Table A-1   Recommended AED Protocol**

**Check Pulse**

If no pulse . . . Do CPR until AED is attached.

**Analyze Rhythm**

If shock advised . . . Defibrillate at 200 joules.

**Analyze Rhythm**

If shock advised . . . Defibrillate at 200-300 joules.

**Analyze Rhythm**

If shock advised . . . Defibrillate at 360 joules.

**Recheck Pulse**

If no pulse . . . Do 1 minute of CPR and recheck pulse.
If still no pulse . . . Repeat analysis and set of 3 shocks at 360 joules as indicated.

**Recheck Pulse**

If no pulse . . . Do 1 minute of CPR and recheck pulse.
If still no pulse . . . Repeat analysis and set of 3 shocks at 360 joules as indicated.

**Recheck Pulse**

If still no pulse . . . Continue CPR and prepare to transport.

NOTE: As long as the pulse is absent and the AED still indicates a need to shock, continue repeating sets of 3 shocks to a maximum of 9 total shocks, with 1 minute of CPR between each set. You should be thoroughly familiar with your local operating procedures, which may vary slightly from this table.

---

The number of shocks the AED administers and the energy level for each shock are often preset by the manufacturers. These energy levels range upward from 200 joules to 360 joules. However, the local medical director can modify the device and establish local operating protocols. The American Heart Association has established guidelines to follow when using the AED and include how CPR is to be used as part of the protocol.

In some instances, the heart will *not* require defibrillation. In this case, the device will inform you that no shock is needed. You should recheck the victim's pulse. If it is still absent, resume CPR. If a pulse is present, recheck breathing. If the victim is still not breathing, continue breathing for the victim and monitoring the pulse.

## Precautions

You need to take the following precautions when using an AED:

* Do not use alcohol pads to clean the chest before attaching the pads.
* Do not defibrillate a victim who has a pulse.
* Do not analyze the rhythm or depress the shock button until everyone is clear of the victim.
* Do not analyze the rhythm or defibrillate in a moving vehicle.
* Do not defibrillate a victim who is in water.
* Do not defibrillate a victim lying on a surface, such as sheet metal, that is likely to transfer the electrical energy to others on or in contact with the same surface.
* Do not defibrillate a victim who is less than 12 years old or weighs less than 90 pounds.
* Do not defibrillate a victim who is wearing a nitroglycerine patch on the chest. Remove any patch from the chest and wipe the area clean before attaching the device.

## ◆ ESTABLISHING AN EARLY DEFIBRILLATION PROGRAM

An early defibrillation program must take into account many variables to be fully successful. These variables include—

* The size, age, and location of the populations to be served.
* The numbers of first responders and more advanced personnel being trained.
* The response times of both first responders and more advanced personnel.
* The number of AEDs available.
* Where the AEDs are placed within the community.
* The commitment to the program from the local medical director and EMS personnel.
* State requirements for certification in automated defibrillation.

When these variables are examined, the programs established can better suit the community. For example, if an extremely large number of older adults live in the northeast section of your community, this is where the AED should be placed. This is because it is the area where cardiac arrests are most likely to occur. If you have several AEDs, they should be strategically placed throughout the community so that response times can be reduced and access to defibrillation can be increased, thereby saving more lives.

## ◆ SUMMARY

Automated external defibrillators (AEDs) show great promise in saving the lives of victims of cardiac arrest. To defibrillate a victim of cardiac arrest by using an AED, take the following basic steps:

* Check for the absence of a pulse to determine cardiac arrest.
* Turn on the AED.
* Attach the device to the victim.
* Deliver a shock if indicated.

You must follow local protocols that establish how many shocks are delivered, the energy setting of each shock, and how CPR and other lifesaving measures are used.

Whether using a fully automatic or semiautomatic defibrillator, both are easy to operate and require minimal training and retraining. Strategically placed in a community where the first persons to arrive on the scene are trained in their use, AEDs are a highly valuable emergency resource of great promise in saving the lives of cardiac arrest victims.

# Glossary

## Pronunciation Guide

*The accented syllable in a word is shown in capital letters.*

*river (RIV er)*

*An unmarked vowel that ends a syllable or comprises a syllable has a long sound.*

*silent (SI lent)*

*A long vowel in a syllable ending in a consonant is marked ‾.*

*snowflake (SNO flāk)*

*An unmarked vowel in a syllable that ends with a consonant has a short sound.*

*sister (SIS ter)*

*A short vowel that comprises a syllable or ends a syllable is marked ˘.*

*decimal (DES ĭ mal)*

*The sound of the letter **a** in an unaccented syllable is spelled **ah**.*

*ahead (ah HED)*

---

**Abandonment:** Ending care of an ill or injured person without that person's consent or without ensuring that someone with equal or greater training will continue that care.

**Abdominal thrusts:** A technique for unblocking an obstructed airway by giving forceful pushes to the abdomen.

**Advanced cardiac life support (ACLS):** Techniques and treatments designed for use with victims of cardiac emergencies.

**AIDS (acquired immune deficiency syndrome):** A condition caused by the human immunodeficiency virus (HIV), which destroys the body's ability to fight infection.

**Airborne transmission:** The transmission of a disease by inhaling infected droplets that become airborne when an infected person coughs or sneezes.

**Airway:** The pathway for air from the mouth and nose to the lungs.

**Airway obstruction:** A blockage of the airway that prevents air from reaching a person's lungs.

**Alveoli (al VE o li):** Tiny air sacs in the lungs where gases and waste are exchanged between the lungs and the blood.

**Anaphylactic (an ah fĭ LAK tik) shock:** A severe allergic reaction in which air passages may swell and restrict breathing; a form of shock.

**Anaphylaxis (an ah fĭ LAK sis):** *see* Anaphylactic shock.

**Anaphylaxis kit:** A container that holds the medication and any necessary equipment used to prevent or counteract anaphylactic shock.

**Anatomical obstruction:** The blockage of the airway by an anatomical structure such as the tongue.

**Angina (an JI nah) pectoris (pek TO ris):** Chest pain that comes and goes at different times; commonly associated with cardiovascular disease.

**Antibiotics (an ti bi OT iks):** Medicines prescribed to help the body fight bacterial infections.

**Antibodies (AN tĭ bod ez):** Infection-fighting proteins released by white blood cells.

**Arteries (AR ter ēz):** The large blood vessels that carry oxygen-rich blood from the heart to all parts of the body.

**Ashen:** A grayish color that darker skin becomes when it turns pale.

**Aspiration (as pĭ RA shun):** Taking blood, vomit, saliva, or other foreign material into the lungs.

**Asthma:** A condition that narrows the air passages and makes breathing difficult.

**Asystole (ah SIS to le):** The stopping of all electrical activity in the heart.

**Atherosclerosis (ath er o skle RO sis):** A form of cardiovascular disease marked by a narrowing of the arteries in the heart and other parts of the body.

**Automatic external defibrillator (de FIB rĭ la tor) (AED):** An automatic device used to recognize a heart rhythm that requires a shock and either delivers the shock or prompts the rescuer to deliver it.

**Bacteria (bac TE re ah):** One-celled microorganisms that may cause infections.

**Bag-valve-mask (BVM) resuscitator:** A hand-held ventilation device, consisting of a self-inflating bag, a one-way valve, and a face mask; can be used with or without supplemental oxygen.

**Biological death:** The irreversible damage caused by the death of brain cells.

**Body substance isolation (BSI):** An infection control strategy that considers all body substances as potentially infectious.

**Body system:** A group of organs and other structures working together to carry out specific functions.

**Brachial (BRA ke al) artery:** A large artery located in the upper arm.

**Brain:** The center of the nervous system that controls all body functions.

**Breathing devices:** Devices used to help with ventilation.

**Breathing emergency:** A situation in which breathing is so impaired that life is threatened.

**Bronchi (BRONG ki):** The air passages that lead from the trachea to the lungs.

**Capillaries (KAP i ler ēz):** Tiny blood vessels linking arteries and veins that transfer oxygen and other nutrients from the blood to all body cells and remove waste products.

**Carbon dioxide:** A colorless, odorless gas; a waste product of respiration.

**Cardiac (KAR de ak) arrest:** A condition in which the heart has stopped or beats too irregularly or too weakly to pump blood effectively.

**Cardiac emergencies:** Sudden illnesses involving the heart.

**Cardiopulmonary (kar de o PUL mo ner e) resuscitation (re sus ĭ TA shun) (CPR):** A technique that combines rescue breathing and chest compressions for a victim whose breathing and heart have stopped.

**Cardiovascular (kar de o VAS ku lar) disease:** A disease of the heart and blood vessels; commonly known as heart disease.

**Carotid arteries:** Arteries located in the neck that supply blood to the head and neck.

**Case law:** A law based on judicial decisions (cases) rather than statutes, which are enacted by legislatures.

**Cells:** The basic units of all living tissue.

**Chest thrusts:** Forceful pushes on the chest; delivered to a person with an obstructed airway in an attempt to expel any foreign object blocking the airway.

**Cholesterol (ko LES ter ol):** A fatty substance made by the body and found in certain foods.

**Circulatory cycle:** The flow of blood in the body: oxygen-rich blood flows through the arteries and oxygen-poor blood flows through the veins.

**Circulatory (SER ku lah tor e) system:** A group of organs and other structures that carry oxygen-rich blood and other nutrients throughout the body and remove waste.

**Citizen responder:** Someone who recognizes an emergency and decides to help; the first link in the emergency medical services (EMS) system.

**Clinical death:** The condition in which the heart stops beating and breathing stops.

**Complete airway obstruction:** A completely blocked airway.

**Confidentiality:** Protecting a victim's privacy by not revealing any personal information you learn about the victim except to law enforcement personnel or EMS personnel caring for the victim.

**Consciousness:** The state of being aware of one's self and one's surroundings.

**Consent:** Permission to provide care given by an ill or injured person to a rescuer.

**Contraction:** The pumping action of the heart.

**Coronary arteries:** Blood vessels that supply the heart muscle with oxygen-rich blood.

**Cricoid cartilage:** A ring-shaped cartilage in the neck.

**Croup:** A viral infection that causes swelling of the tissues below the vocal cords; a common childhood illness.

**Cyanosis (si ah NO sis):** A blue discoloration of the skin and membranes of the mouth and eyes, resulting from a lack of oxygen in the blood.

**Defibrillation (de fib ri LA shun):** An electric shock administered to correct a life-threatening heart rhythm.

**Defibrillator (de FIB ri la tor):** A device that sends an electric shock through the chest to the heart.

**Dentures:** A set of false teeth.

**Diaphragm (DI ah fram):** A dome-shaped muscle that aids breathing and separates the chest from the abdomen.

**Direct contact transmission:** The transmission of a disease by touching an infected person's body fluids.

**Disease transmission:** The passage of a disease from one person to another.

**Drowning:** Death by suffocation when submerged in water.

**Drug:** Any substances other than food intended to affect the functions of the body.

**Duty to act:** A legal responsibility of certain people to provide a reasonable standard of emergency care; may be required by case law, statute, or job description.

**Electrical burn:** A burn caused by an electrical source such as an electrical appliance or lightning.

**Electrocardiogram (e lek tro KAR de o gram) (ECG):** The movement of the electrical impulses down the pathway, shown as a tracing on a screen.

**Embolism (EM bo lizm):** A sudden blockage of a blood vessel by a traveling clot or other material, such as fat or air.

**Emergency action principles (EAPs):** Four steps to guide a rescuer's actions in any emergency.

**Emergency medical services (EMS) system:** A network of community resources and medical personnel that provides emergency care to victims of injury or sudden illness.

**Emergency medical technician (EMT):** Someone who has successfully completed a state-approved emergency medical technician training program; different levels of EMTs include paramedics at the highest level.

**Emergency move:** Moving a victim before completing care; only performed if the victim is in immediate danger.

**Emphysema (em fi SE mah):** A disease in which the lungs lose their ability to exchange carbon dioxide and oxygen effectively.

**Epiglottis (ep i GLOT is):** The flap of tissue that covers the trachea to keep food and liquid out of the lungs.

**Epiglottitis:** A bacterial infection that causes a severe inflammation of the epiglottis.

**Esophagus (e SOF ah gus):** The tube leading from the mouth to the stomach.

**Exhale:** To breathe air out of the lungs.

**Finger sweep:** A technique used to remove foreign material from a victim's airway.

**First responder:** A person trained in emergency care who may be called on to provide such care as a routine part of his or her job; often the first trained professional to respond to emergencies.

**Gastric distention:** Air in the stomach.

**Good Samaritan laws:** Laws that protect people who willingly give emergency care without accepting anything in return.

**Head-tilt/chin-lift:** A technique for opening the airway.

**Heart:** A fist-sized muscular organ that circulates blood throughout the body.

**Heart attack:** A sudden illness involving the death of heart muscle tissue when it does not receive enough oxygen-rich blood.

**Heimlich maneuver:** A technique used to clear the airway of a choking victim; *see* Abdominal thrusts.

**Hepatitis (hep ah TI tis):** A viral infection of the liver; forms include hepatitis A and hepatitis B.

**Hepatitis A:** A type of hepatitis that is transmitted by contact with food or other products contaminated by the stool of an infected person; also called infectious hepatitis.

**Hepatitis B:** A type of hepatitis that is transmitted by sexual contact and blood-to-blood contact; also called serum hepatitis.

**Herpes (HER pez):** A viral infection that causes eruptions of the skin and mucous membranes.

**High efficiency particulate air-particulate respirator (HEPA-PR):** A protective breathing device containing a high efficiency air filter that prevents transmission of certain airborne infections.

**HIV (human immunodeficiency virus):** The virus that causes AIDS.

**Hyperventilation:** Breathing that is faster than normal.

**Hypothermia:** A life-threatening condition in which the body's warming mechanisms fail to maintain normal body temperature, and the entire body cools.

**Immune system:** The body's group of responses for fighting disease.

**Immunization (im u ni ZA shun):** The introduction of a specific substance containing weakened or killed pathogens into the body to build resistance to a specific infection.

**Implied consent:** A legal concept assuming that persons who are unconscious, or so severely injured or ill that they cannot respond, would consent to receive emergency care.

**Indirect contact transmission:** The transmission of a disease by touching a contaminated object.

**Infant:** A child up to 1 year of age.

**Infection:** A condition caused by disease-producing microorganisms, also called pathogens or germs, in the body.

**Infectious disease:** A communicable disease.

**Informed (actual) consent:** Permission the victim, parent, or guardian gives the rescuer to provide care. This consent requires the rescuer to explain his or her level of training, what the rescuer thinks is wrong, and the care the rescuer intends to give.

**Inhalant:** A substance, such as a medication, that a person inhales to counteract or prevent a specific condition; a substance inhaled to produce an intoxicating effect.

**Inhale:** To breathe in.

**Larynx (LAR ingks):** A part of the airway connecting the pharynx with the trachea; commonly called the "voice box."

**Level of consciousness (LOC):** A person's state of awareness, ranging from being fully alert to unconscious.

**Living will:** A legal document stating that an individual does not wish to be resuscitated or be further kept alive by mechanical means.

**Lungs:** A pair of organs in the chest that provides the mechanism for taking oxygen in and removing carbon dioxide during breathing.

**Mechanical obstruction:** The blockage of the airway by a foreign object such as a small toy or food.

**Medication:** A drug given to prevent or correct the effects of a disease or condition or otherwise enhance mental or physical welfare.

**Membrane:** A thin sheet of tissue that covers a structure or lines a cavity such as the mouth or nose.

**Meningitis (men in JI tis):** An inflammation of the brain or spinal cord caused by a viral or bacterial infection.

**Minor:** A person who has not reached full legal age.

**Multi-drug resistant TB:** A strain of tuberculosis that is resistant to certain drugs commonly used to treat tuberculosis.

**Muscle:** Tissue that lengthens and shortens to create movement.

**Near-drowning:** A situation in which a person who has been submerged in water survives.

**Negligence:** The failure to provide the level of care a person of similar training would provide, thereby causing injury or damage to another.

**Nerve:** A part of the nervous system that sends impulses to and from the brain and all other body parts.

**Nervous system:** A group of organs and other structures that regulates all body functions.

**Normal sinus rhythm:** A regular heart rhythm that occurs within a normal rate and without unusual variations.

**Organ:** A collection of similar tissues acting together to perform specific body functions.

**Oxygen:** A tasteless, colorless, odorless gas necessary to sustain life.

**Paramedics:** Highly specialized EMTs.

**Partial airway obstruction:** An incomplete blockage of the airway.

**Pathogen (PATH o jen):** A disease-causing agent; also called a microorganism or germ.

**Personal protective equipment (PPE):** Specialized clothing or equipment worn for protection from a hazard.

**Pharynx (FAR ingks):** A part of the airway formed by the back of the nose and throat.

**Primary survey:** A check for conditions that are an immediate threat to a victim's life.

**Protocols:** Standardized methods.

**Public safety personnel:** People employed in a governmental system who are required to respond to and assist with a medical emergency; includes police, fire fighters, and ambulance personnel.

**Pulse:** The beat felt in arteries with each contraction of the heart.

**Radial pulse:** The pulse felt in the wrist.

**Refusal of care:** The declining of care by a victim; the victim has the right to refuse the care of anyone who responds to an emergency scene.

**Rehabilitation:** The restoration of a victim to his or her previous state of health.

**Rescue breathing:** A technique of breathing for a nonbreathing victim.

**Respiration (res pi RA shun):** The breathing process of the body that takes in oxygen and eliminates carbon dioxide.

**Respiratory (re SPI rah to re *or* RES pah rah tor e) system:** A group of organs and other structures that bring air into the body and remove wastes through a process called breathing, or respiration.

**Respiratory arrest:** A condition in which breathing has stopped.

**Respiratory distress:** A condition in which breathing is difficult.

**Resuscitation mask:** A pliable, dome-shaped device that fits over a person's mouth and nose, used to assist with rescue breathing.

**Ribs:** Bones that attach to the spine and sternum and protect the heart and lungs.

**Risk factors:** Conditions or behaviors that increase the chance that a person will develop a disease.

**Saturated fat:** Fat derived from animal products; a solid at room temperature.

**Secondary survey:** A check for injuries or conditions that could become life-threatening if not cared for.

**Signs:** Any observable evidence of injury or illness, such as bleeding or an unusually pale skin color.

**Spinal cord:** A bundle of nerves extending from the base of the skull to the lower back; protected by the spinal column.

**Spine:** A series of bones (vertebrae) that surround and protect the spinal cord; also called the backbone.

**Standard of care:** The minimal standard and quality of care expected of an emergency care provider.

**Statute:** A written law; a law enacted by a legislature.

**Sternum (STER num):** The long flat bone in the middle of the front of the rib cage; also called the breastbone.

**Stoma:** An opening in the front of the neck through which a person whose larynx has been removed breathes.

**Stroke:** A disruption of blood flow to a part of the brain that causes permanent damage; also called a cerebrovascular accident (CVA).

**Sudden death:** The occurrence of cardiac arrest without any prior sign of heart attack.

**Supplemental oxygen:** Additional oxygen provided to help resuscitate a person.

**Symptoms:** Something the victim tells you about his or her condition, such as, "My head hurts," or "I am dizzy."

**Tissue:** A collection of similar cells acting together to perform specific body functions.

**Trachea (TRA ke ah):** A tube leading from the upper airway to the lungs; also called the windpipe.

**Trauma:** Physical injury caused by shock, pressure, or violence.

**Trauma center:** A medical facility specially equipped and staffed to give immediate emergency care to victims of trauma.

**Tuberculosis (tu ber ku LO sis) (TB):** A respiratory disease caused by a bacteria.

**Universal precautions:** Safety measures taken to prevent occupational-risk exposure to blood or other body fluids containing visible blood.

**Vaccine:** A medical substance containing killed or weakened microorganisms that is introduced into the body to prevent, kill, or treat a disease.

**Vector transmission:** The transmission of a disease by an animal or insect bite.

**Veins:** Blood vessels that carry oxygen-poor blood from all parts of the body to the heart.

**Ventilation:** The process of providing oxygen to the lungs through rescue breathing or by other means.

**Ventricular (ven TRIK u lar) fibrillation (fi bri LA shun) (V-fib):** A state of totally disorganized electrical activity in the heart, resulting in the quivering (fibrillation) of the ventricles.

**Ventricular tachycardia (tak e KAR de ah):** A heart rate so fast that the heart is unable to pump blood properly.

**Virus (VI rus):** A disease-causing agent, or pathogen, that requires another organism to live and reproduce.

**Vital organs:** Organs whose functions are essential to life, including the brain, heart, and lungs.

**Xiphoid (ZI foid):** An arrow-shaped piece of hard tissue at the lowest point of the sternum.

# Index

# MISSION OF THE AMERICAN RED CROSS

The American Red Cross, a humanitarian organization led by volunteers and guided by its Congressional Charter and the Fundamental Principles of the International Red Cross Movement, will provide relief to victims of disaster and help people prevent, prepare for, and respond to emergencies.

# ABOUT THE AMERICAN RED CROSS

To support the mission of the American Red Cross, over 1.3 million paid and volunteer staff serve in some 1,600 chapters and blood centers throughout the United States and its territories and on military installations around the world. Supported by the resources of a national organization, they form the largest volunteer service and educational force in the nation. They serve families and communities through blood services, disaster relief and preparedness education, services to military family members in crisis, and health and safety education.

The American Red Cross provides consistent, reliable education and training in injury and illness prevention and emergency care, providing training to nearly 16 million people each year in first aid, CPR, swimming, water safety, and HIV/AIDS education.

All of these essential services are made possible by the voluntary services, blood and tissue donations, and financial support of the American people.

# FUNDAMENTAL PRINCIPLES OF THE INTERNATIONAL RED CROSS AND RED CRESCENT MOVEMENT

HUMANITY

IMPARTIALITY

NEUTRALITY

INDEPENDENCE

VOLUNTARY SERVICE

UNITY

UNIVERSALITY